Agnes Warner and the Nursing Sisters of the Great War

The New Brunswick Military Heritage Series, Volume 15

Agnes Warner and the
NURSING SISTERS
of the Great War

Shawna M. Quinn

GOOSE LANE EDITIONS and
THE NEW BRUNSWICK MILITARY HERITAGE PROJECT

Edited by Brent Wilson and Barry Norris.
Front cover images courtesy of Library and Archives Canada: LAC-PA-002562 (top), LAC-PA-006783 (bottom).
Back cover illustration entitled "Sister," courtesy of Canadian War Museum: CWM 19700046-012, portrait of Agnes Warner courtesy of *My Beloved Poilus*, uniform courtesy of CWM 19590034-002.
Cover and interior page design by Jaye Haworth.
Art direction by Julie Scriver.
Printed in Canada on FSC certified paper.
10 9 8 7 6 5 4 3 2 1

Library and Archives Canada Cataloguing in Publication

Quinn, Shawna M., 1977-
   Agnes Warner and the Nursing Sisters of the Great War / Shawna M. Quinn.

(New Brunswick military heritage series; v. 15)
Co-published by: New Brunswick Military Heritage Project.
Includes bibliographical references and index.
ISBN 978-0-86492-633-3

1. Warner, Agnes. 2. World War, 1914-1918 — Medical care — Canada.
3. World War, 1914-1918 — Personal narratives, Canadian.
4. Nurses — New Brunswick — Biography.
I. New Brunswick Military Heritage Project
II. Title. III. Series: New Brunswick military heritage series; v. 15

D629.C2Q56 2010   940.4'7571510922   C2010-904375-8

Goose Lane Editions acknowledges the financial support of the Canada Council for the Arts, the Government of Canada through the Book Publishing Industry Development Program (BPIDP), and the New Brunswick Department of Wellness, Culture and Sport for its publishing activities.

Goose Lane Editions
Suite 330, 500 Beaverbrook Court
Fredericton, New Brunswick
CANADA E3B 5X4
www.gooselane.com

New Brunswick Military Heritage Project
The Brigadier Milton F. Gregg, VC,
Centre for the Study of War and Society
University of New Brunswick
PO Box 4400
Fredericton, New Brunswick
CANADA E3B 5A3
www.unb.ca/nbmhp

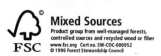

Mixed Sources
Product group from well-managed forests, controlled sources and recycled wood or fiber
www.fsc.org Cert no. SW-COC-000952
© 1996 Forest Stewardship Council
FSC

Contents

Chapter One

"I Have Been There, Too"

Former Canadian army nursing sister Katherine Wilson-Simmie was nearly eighty years old when she finally undertook to publish an account of her wartime nursing experience for a wider readership beyond her immediate family. She began by referring to stories of danger and soldiers' bravery, knowing that these accounts, told by the men who lived them, had continued to capture the imagination of Canadians like her children and grandchildren throughout the six decades since the Great War. But she also felt that the soldiers' accounts "tended to romanticize things," and wondered aloud why no books had been written by Canadian army nursing sisters. There were many male authors writing about important First World War campaigns. She said, "Well, I have been there, too."

Katherine Wilson-Simmie's recollections, published in 1981 as *Lights Out! A Canadian Nursing Sister's Tale*, is exceptional among Canadian First World War nurses' accounts for being one of only a handful to have been published after the war, and its belatedness is noteworthy. The First World War was a global conflict such as no one had ever seen. It pulverized untold hectares of landscape, killed millions of soldiers and civilians, and gripped much of Canada with a fervent patriotism, drawing the nation's resources and humanity into unknown dangers across the Atlantic. As Canadians mobilized to fight "Might" with "Right," women were there, too. On the home front, they replaced absent men in munitions factories, farms, and other areas of employment formerly closed to women, while overseas they served in non-combatant and traditionally feminine roles. There were opportunities for women to help by cooking and performing other supportive work in England and elsewhere, but if they wanted a heady brush with all the urgency and immediacy of combat, the only accepted female contribution offering anything close to the frontline experience was nursing. The need for trained nurses was great, and well over three thousand Canadian women enthusiastically answered the call, suppressing whatever vague premonitions they had of the difficulties that lay ahead.

Most of these nurses would return home to Canada after the war to resume or re-create their lives. And that's when these women — who had seen extraordinary sights, suffered abysmal conditions, and mended so many shattered bodies — fell silent about what they had experienced. But not immediately, since theirs was an adventure that few Canadian women could have imagined and all wanted to hear about. Before they could vanish altogether into their former routines, these returning heroes found themselves drawn into a whirlwind of triumphant "welcome home" receptions, during which they recounted their stories to transfixed audiences and accepted their accolades with appropriate humility. Paraphrases of these lectures survive in the limited columns of local newspapers, but how many of the nurses' own words made it to publication?

Very few, in fact, but it was not for lack of prompting. In fall 1920, Margaret Macdonald, who had been wartime Matron-in-Chief of the Canadian Army Medical Corps (C.A.M.C.) Nursing Service, wrote to former nursing sisters asking for their reminiscences to include in a "full account of the conspicuously distinguished work of this corps." She hoped each of the twenty-five hundred recipients of the letter would contribute a "characteristic incident, a telling photograph or authentic circumstance of historical value that came under [her] personal observation." Macdonald's request yielded a meagre eight responses. Of these, some respectfully declined to contribute, while others apologized for having nothing of importance to offer or recounted a second-hand story they'd heard from a soldier. Why such reticence on the part of nurses who were every bit the "eyewitnesses" of war's extremes that soldiers were?

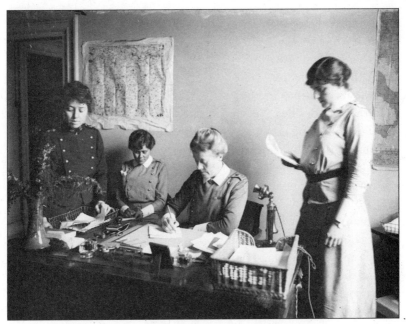

Office of Matron-in-Chief Margaret Macdonald. LAC-PA-5230

Perhaps the phrase "of historical value" made many nurses doubt their personal observations could be worthy of inclusion in a national history of the Great War. Perhaps they felt it immodestly out of character for nurses to publicize their working experience and achievements, an attitude reinforced by wartime propaganda and earlier representations of nurses as discreet, self-effacing "angels of mercy." Macdonald's biographer, Susan Mann, suggests that, besides these other grounds for discretion, nurses had a professional obligation to maintain a quiet, therapeutic atmosphere around the wounded and to protect their privacy when off duty. Even more urgently, silence was a wartime expedient: under the constraints of War Office censorship, nurses had to be circumspect about the details of their work, and the habit of self-censorship they adopted lasted well beyond the Armistice. And if there weren't external pressures enough for nurses to downplay their experiences, there were deep-rooted, private motives. Women who had seen horrors beyond words naturally shrank from the heart-wrenching task of serving them up in print to an uninitiated, if sympathetic, audience.

A few Canadian nursing sisters, however, did put pen to paper after the war. Besides Wilson-Simmie's *Light's Out!*, there was Mabel Clint's penetrating account of her service in France, England, and the Mediterranean island of Lemnos entitled *Our Bit: Memories of War Service by a Canadian Nursing Sister* (1934). Both of these authors, though, waited many years before publishing their accounts. One of the earliest offerings was from C.A.M.C. Nursing Sister Constance Bruce, who in 1918 informally published a lighthearted but often poignant narrative called *Humour in Tragedy.* This short work is witty and lively, illustrated with tongue-in-cheek drawings of nurses in high action — veils blowing out behind them like cones as they got up to good-natured tricks, enduring the discomforts of camp life (such as missing laundry or swarming flies), and gamely enjoying the novelties of local culture, all with an endearing readiness to laugh, cry, and *experience.* It is interesting that the foreword of this little book, written by Lord Beaverbrook, implies that the reader should treat it as a personalized "peep behind the scenes" in the absence of an official C.A.M.C. history, which was then being compiled by Sir Andrew Macphail under commission of the Department of National Defence and would not be published until 1925. In the meantime, Beaverbrook assured the reader that

> The official record of this branch of the Canadian service
> is in able hands, but this book of Miss Constance Bruce
> …is a very unofficial and delightful tale of the adventures
> of No. 1 Canadian Stationary Hospital in France, at
> Lemnos, at Cairo and at Salonica…I am certain the book
> will commend itself not only to all Canadians, but the
> wider public of the British Empire, which is only realizing
> slowly the steadfastness of our women in their adventures
> in the greatest adventure in the world.

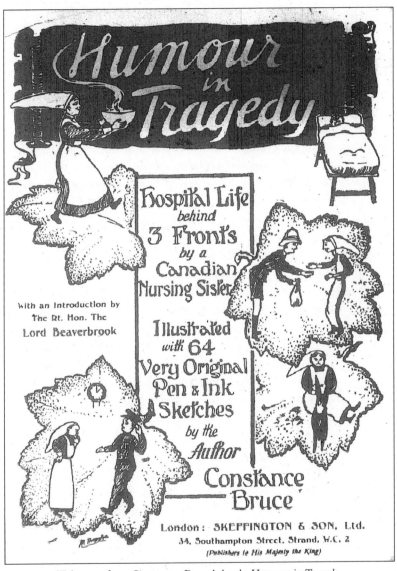

Title page from Constance Bruce's book, *Humour in Tragedy*.

While nurses' stories may have brought women's contributions to light and captured human interest, they would not find a place in the "official" record. Perhaps if more than a handful of her charges had answered Matron Macdonald's call for contributions, her volume might have taken its intended place beside Macphail's among the histories of Canada's role in the Great War. But she did not complete the project. Instead, her effort survives as six pages in Macphail's chapter on "The Ancillary Services," briefly surveying the evolution of the military nursing service in Canada and devoid of any personalized observations from nurses. The official history itself, moreover, does not dare to portray the war through nurses' eyes. Take, for instance, the way it follows the wounded man's progress through various stages of medical aid, beginning with the moment he is hit. The author describes that instant as an experience of painless "wonder." The man on the stretcher then views the ensuing rush to the casualty clearing station with "apathy and unconcern" — but still no pain. It is not until he reaches the base hospital that pain hits the soldier with all its force, whereafter it becomes "atrocious and had best not be spoken of even in a history of military medicine. To witness this suffering which they could so imperfectly allay was the *continuous and appalling experience of the nurses* at the front and at the base." Bearing witness to unspeakable pain was the nurses' predominant experience, yet even the C.A.M.C.'s historian draws the curtain on this phase of suffering rather than attempt to depict it, and abruptly ends the chapter there. Behind the curtain, nurses continued to work.

Where can a reader go, then, for nurses' personal accounts? Fortunately, Canadian women working overseas were highly motivated to record their experiences in private diaries — some terse and pragmatic, others literary and rhetorical. Because of their personal and solitary nature, unpublished diaries can be difficult to find. But a rare few have been published, such as those of Ella Mae Bongard, edited by her son Eric Scott, in *Nobody Ever Wins A War* and Nova Scotia nurse Clare Gass, edited and introduced by historian Susan Mann, in *The War Diary of Clare Gass, 1915-1918*.

Canadian nursing sisters on active service far from home were also motivated to keep communion with their loved ones through frequent letters. Like diaries, many of these letters remain out of reach in private collections, but in their time they had a wider distribution than diaries. They were circulated among family and friends and sometimes even found their way into the columns of regional newspapers alongside soldiers' letters from the trenches. On much rarer occasions, friends might collaborate to gather a nurse's letters together and publish them in an effort to raise awareness and funds for her continuing work. It is in this latter way that we come to possess Nursing Sister Agnes Warner's wartime letters published under the title *My Beloved Poilus,* an enduring expression of one New Brunswick nurse's devotion to the people of wartorn France and Belgium. Though Warner's journey to the front lines differs from that of other Canadian nurses in significant ways since she did not serve with the Canadian army, her trajectory from nursing student to Edwardian private-duty nurse to nurse under fire has much in common with that of her "sisters."

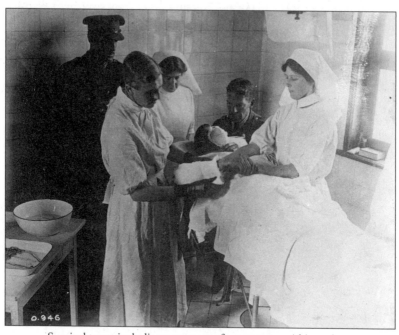

Surgical team, including a nurse, perform surgery within an hour
of the patient's being wounded. CWM 19920085-102

Chapter Two

New Brunswick Nurses Go to War

In 1914, the occupation of "nursing" as we know it today, with all the hard-won trappings of a genuine profession, was relatively young. Certainly, women had been providing medical care for their families and communities for centuries, but this work was not recognized as professional, skilled work. Rather, it was considered domestic, innate, and inherently feminine. Women were predisposed to care for and heal others as a result of their "natural calling," not by virtue of any special training, knowledge, or certification. Those who nursed full time tended to be members of religious orders or were effectively domestic servants, caring for ailing people in private homes or central hospitals that served the poor. Gains famously made by Florence Nightingale in the mid-nineteenth century sparked a vision of occupational rigour that moved pioneers on several continents to begin establishing nursing schools and pushing for occupational standards. But even as late as the 1870s, women working in North American urban hospitals typically were untrained, working class, and accorded lowly status by both the medical profession they supported and society at large. Nursing under these conditions held little appeal for promising young middle-class Maritime women, to say nothing of their parents.

But by the time Margaret Macdonald, Agnes Warner, and the other Canadian women who would eventually serve in the Great War first considered nursing as a career, perceptions had changed. Thanks to the persistence of the pioneer female administrators of hospital-based nursing schools in applying Nightingale's model, the standards of classroom and on-the-job training had risen sharply in the 1880s and 1890s, and along with them the expectation of decorous and professional conduct. An exacting and military-like discipline governed most training schools, where first-year probationer nurses endured long days cleaning their wards and feeding and bathing patients before they were accepted into the intermediate ranks and given ever-more sensitive responsibilities with patients. Academic study filled the hours between gruelling shifts on the hospital floor. By the turn of the century, programs in Canadian and US hospitals had turned out multiple classes of proud graduates for whom a career in nursing meant a respectable and fulfilling profession that not only paid good wages, but also offered an unusual opportunity for administrative power and personal autonomy.

Not unexpectedly, this transition left many behind, for one of the drivers of this push for professionalism was the elimination of uncertified competition. The survival of the educated, professional nurse depended on replacing the notion that *any* woman could be a nurse with the conviction that only the brightest, the formally trained, and the socially upstanding could be entrusted with the job. Partly in reaction to the longstanding perception of nurses as disreputable, even morally suspect, nursing leaders promoted a new image of nursing school graduates who came from "good" families and whose dedication to caring for others had carried them through the fires of a rigorous training program. It wasn't difficult for a probationer to get herself ejected for showing poor aptitude or violating the strict behavioural code. Nursing programs thus became more and more elitist, even more so in Canada and the United States than elsewhere.

This gleaming new image became an important part of nurses' participation in the First World War. The graduate nurse's certificate served as an endorsement of her character and her ticket to independent adventures both at home and overseas. With Britain's declaration of war against Germany in early August 1914, a move that automatically involved Canada, the possibilities for service abroad exploded. After that point, provided she met the qualifications for training and age (the minimum age varied from twenty-one to twenty-five years), the trained Canadian nurse could offer her services and be readily accepted in Britain, where administrators were busy setting up an International Nursing Corps and where the Queen Alexandra's Imperial Military Nursing Service (Q.A.I.M.N.S.) had been staffing British military hospitals efficiently for ten years. Or she could sign up with various branches of the Red Cross in virtually any country touched by the growing conflict. Many Canadian women made it overseas through their own arrangements and on their own dime, joining whatever organization could put them to work.

As the scale of the fight surpassed all imagination, it quickly became apparent to the Canadian military that Britain needed more than Canada's troops on the front line; medical personnel were also in great demand, and that included nurses. Before August 1914, there were only five nurses in the Permanent Army Medical Corps in Canada and some fifty-seven on the reserve Army Nursing Service list. There was no difficulty finding new recruits. Throughout August, applications from graduate nurses poured in by the hundreds. From these, an initial one hundred trained nurses were to be selected; inoculated; hastily trained for army service (if they were not army-trained already); outfitted with a sky-blue work uniform, navy wool dress uniform, and camp kit; and sent off with the staffs of two general hospitals that accompanied the Canadian Expeditionary Force (C.E.F.) to Europe in those early months of the war.

At least nine nurses from Saint John, New Brunswick, went with this first contingent to work in the No. 1 General Hospital, commanded by Colonel (Dr.) Murray MacLaren of Saint John. Among them were Miss Grace Domville and Margaret Parks, who was actually a medical doctor in civilian life. No female doctors or male nurses were recruited, though a few female doctors circumvented the red tape and cooperatively founded special non-military hospitals, like Saint John doctor Catherine Travis's baby hospital in Serbia. Moreover, no female staff went with the stationary hospitals and casualty clearing stations of the C.E.F. in the first contingent. These hospitals, located closer to the front, were in danger of enemy fire and their personnel had to be ready to evacuate at a moment's notice. The larger general hospitals, though, were accommodated in abandoned schools, donated mansions, or other reasonably suitable buildings in safer zones.

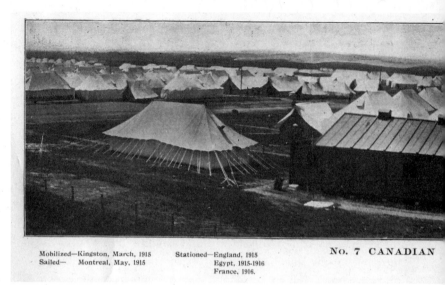

Mobilized—Kingston, March, 1915 Stationed—England, 1915 No. 7 CANADIAN
Sailed— Montreal, May, 1915 Egypt, 1915-1916
France, 1916.

No. 7 Canadian General Hospital. Queen's University Picture Collection V28 Mil-Hosp-10

Before conditions convinced military authorities of the need to install nurses at advanced hospitals, a wounded soldier had to pass through several gruelling stages before he even saw a nurse. From the place he fell, he would have to wait for stretcher bearers to find him under cover of darkness and take him to the nearest first aid post, or try to crawl there by himself. From there he might be sent to an advanced dressing station or be conveyed by horse-drawn or motorized ambulance over appalling roads to a main dressing station to have his condition classified. If gravely wounded, he might be operated on immediately, then sent further back to the casualty clearing station as soon as he could be moved. If the wound was less serious, he would have an opportunity to recuperate somewhat before returning to the front. Casualty clearing stations (C.C.S.s) were set up on railway sidings less than five miles from the front. Earlier in the war, their staff chiefly dressed wounds and loaded casualties onto trains bound for larger hospitals in the rear: the (misleadingly named) stationary hospitals, with up to five hundred beds but designed to be mobile, or the

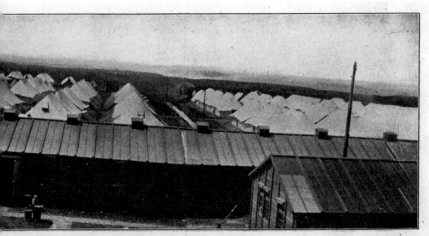

HOSPITAL (QUEEN'S).

LT.-COL. ETHERINGTON, C.M.G.,
O.C.

MISS B. WILLOUGHBY,
Matron.

larger general hospitals, with a thousand to fifteen hundred beds and as many as a hundred nurses. Before long, however, C.C.S.s evolved into advanced surgical hospitals that provided life-saving operations before wounds became infected beyond hope. An obvious need for nurses trumped any lingering misgivings about putting women in harm's way, and before long select nurses held coveted positions in the casualty clearing stations, too. Duty so close to the firing line demanded the utmost efficiency — the best of the best — and nurses considered it a personal honour to be assigned to this work.

Back home, Canadian nurses continued to sign up in droves for active service. Applications flooded the desk of Matron-in-Chief Margaret Macdonald — too many to process, never mind accept, in 1914. As the front settled into a static line of trenches stretching from the Belgian coast to the Swiss border and casualty numbers mounted, the demand for Canadian nurses grew steadily but still could not keep pace with the number of applicants waiting anxiously to find out if they'd be next to

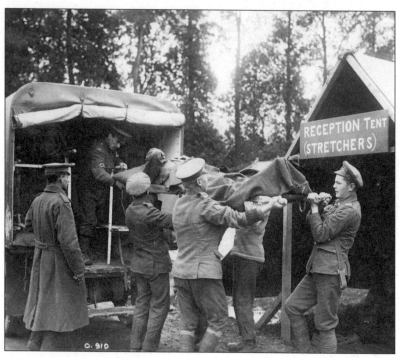

Unloading a stretcher carrying a wounded soldier from a truck to a reception tent at a Canadian casualty clearing station. CWM 19920044-811

steam across the Atlantic. Colonel Guy Carleton Jones, head of what was by now called the Canadian Army Medical Corps (C.A.M.C.), did his part to dissuade fair-weather recruits. Addressing a meeting of the Ottawa Graduate Nurses' Association, he sternly warned that "Active service work is extremely severe. A very large proportion of regular nurses are totally unfit, physically and mentally, for it." If his caution gave some women pause, it did not appear to curb interest. And no wonder: with slogans such as "Come on Boys!" and "Your King and Country Need You," Canada was enjoining its young men to enlist and face unknown horrors. For nurses, too, the call to defend civilization resonated loudly

Facing page: Canada Food Board poster targeting housewives.
McGill University WP1.F12.F2

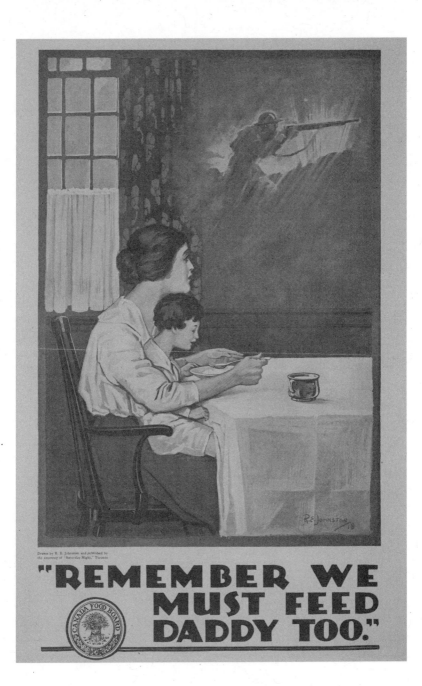

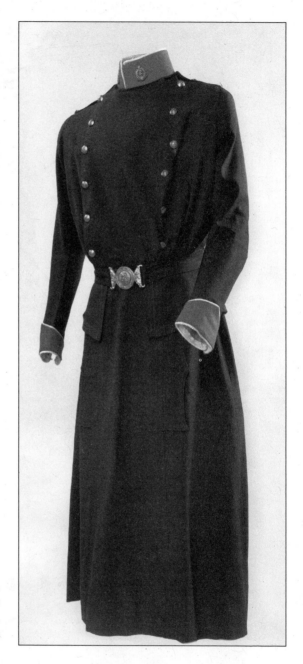

C.A.M.C.
nurse's dress
uniform.
CWM 19590034-002

in both the conscience and the imagination. Here was an opportunity to stand on the same ground as their countrymen and restore them with comfort and healing if they fell — to serve the nation in a way for which nurses were uniquely qualified. There is little doubt that the active service posters targeting Canadian men struck nurses more forcibly than messages pleading women to knit furiously and economize on the home front. What is more, nurses were free to go. The vast majority were unmarried, with an unusual degree of independence and a salary, and although most would never have considered international travel before, the war now facilitated their going and there was nothing standing in their way. Canadian army nurses would see service in England's cities and countryside, France's coastal resort towns, Belgium's villages, scorching eastern Mediterranean islands, and even, for four "fortunate" women, Russia in the midst of revolution. As Canadian soldier recruits rushed overseas with enthusiasm, so did Canadian nurses. One nursing sister put it very plainly in retrospect: "I wanted to be in the Army because I was curious; I wanted to see what it was like." Once contracted, most nurses were locked into service "for the duration" of the war, and only personal illness, daughterly duties (such as those resulting from death or illness in the family), or matrimony could release them. Few nurses traded service for marriage during the war, but it was not unheard of.

For some nurses, the impetus to serve abroad came from a deeply personal need to be physically close to beloved fiancés, friends, and relatives as they struggled in the fight of their lives. Matron Macdonald recognized this motivation as an important one for keeping C.A.M.C. nurses in good spirits, and wherever possible she arranged for her nurses to work near loved ones posted with the C.E.F. For those who had lost dear ones already, the busy-work of nursing offered a way to overcome their private tragedies, feel more worthy of their beloved's sacrifice, and keep from drowning in personal despair.

The call to service also struck a chord with the ideology of their profession. Nurses had always protected individual humans. Now they were called to protect humankind with the angelic self-denial and maternal purity that went hand-in-hand with the ideal of the "true" nurse. Images of mother-nurses bearing angel's wings cradling wounded men figured prominently in recruitment posters on both sides of the Atlantic. Such chaste and noble depictions also reassured families back home who feared the unwholesome effects of globetrotting and army coarseness on their daughters. Nurses themselves reinforced their maternal role by referring to the wounded as "lads" or "boys."

Then there were the perks. Besides the sense of importance that came with participation in active service, which excluded most other women, a C.A.M.C. nursing sister's position came with paid room and board, amounting to about $2.60 per day, and beautiful blue uniforms that earned Canadian nurses the cheery nickname "Bluebirds" and incited envy from grey-clad Imperial and Red Cross nurses everywhere. Canadian nursing sisters loved their C.A.M.C. uniforms. The cornflower blue workday outfit with full white apron and shoulder-length white veil gave them the look of schoolgirls, nuns, or ministering angels — perfectly in keeping with the "Sister" moniker that was a carryover from the days when religious orders did full-time nursing and aptly implied exclusive membership in a carefully guarded club. The darker blue dress uniform boasted two rows of brass buttons, a scarlet-lined cape, and brimmed dress hat. It was altogether a sharp outfit, but one feature of particular significance glinted from the shoulder and distinguished the C.A.M.C. nurse from her British counterparts: the two stars of a lieutenant. For nearly a decade, C.A.M.C. nursing sisters had enjoyed officers' rank: lieutenant for nurses, captain for matrons in charge of hospitals, and major reserved for the matron-in-chief. Army officials justified officers' ranks for nurses (albeit without a command or full commission) on the basis of nurses' social origins, their higher education, and the propriety of elevating them a respectful distance above the rank-and-file soldiers whose bodies they mended. C.A.M.C. historian J. George Adami recognized that the nurses' rank was a somewhat contentious subject when he defended it in 1918:

> While...there are English, Scotch and Irish nursing sisters
> not one whit behind their Canadian sisters in any respect,
> socially, as a body, the nursing profession in Canada has,

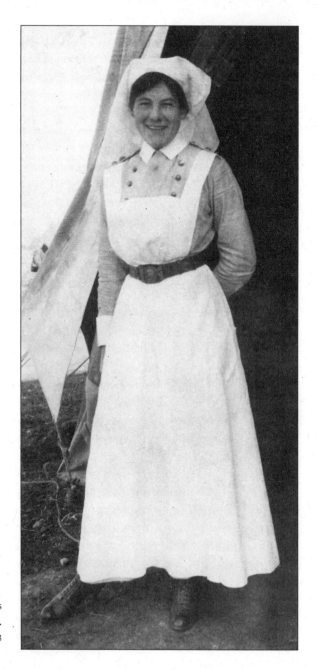

C.A.M.C. nurse's
working uniform.
LAC 1970-163

in the first place, a higher status than it possesses in the old country. It attracts, in general, the daughters of professional men, and those from comfortable households...It is a rule that Canadian Nursing Sisters have had, not a common, but a High School education...And as nurses their training has been very thorough, with fuller courses of lectures on the basal subjects than is usual in Great Britain. As a result, a remarkably large proportion of the matrons of the great hospitals in the United States are of Canadian birth and training. Add to this that the Canadian nurse embarked on her profession is paid on a scale which in Great Britain would be thought extravagant. But then she is thoroughly competent... [I]n this war they have abundantly "made good."

Adami then hastened to uphold the nurses' humility, as if their elevation was more richly deserved because they did not demand it suffragette-style: "It should be emphasized that this step was taken...by the Ministry and Militia Council, not as the result of any agitation by the nursing sisters themselves — in fact, some years before the suffragettes became militant. The experience of the Canadian Army Medical Service has abundantly justified the innovation and proved it to be right and wise."

As lieutenants, Canadian nursing sisters could attend the entertainments hosted by other officers, enjoy relatively comfortable amenities, and claim respect and obedience from orderlies in the military hospitals. Meanwhile, the British army continued to deny rank to nurses in the Q.A.I.M.N.S., itself a non-military organization but still the chief body of nurses supporting Britain's military. Not surprisingly, the issue of rank occasionally fuelled tension between co-working British nurses disdainful of uppity "colonials" and Canadian nurses who resented being treated as inferiors. For the most part, however, working relations between nurses of the two countries were cordial, even warm, as troubling inequalities gave way to mutual purpose.

Some Canadian nurses even donned the uniform of the British

Q.A.I.M.N.S. In September 1916, the Saint John *Daily Telegraph* reported that a new request for two hundred nurses for the Q.A.I.M.N.S. "will no doubt satisfy the desires of a number of trained nurses who wish to get overseas." Sixty-six of these were to come from the Maritime provinces, and interested women applied at the Royal Victoria Hospital in Montreal. Contracts were for one year, renewable, or for the duration of the war; return passage and uniforms were provided.

❖❖

Other important routes to the front arose besides the C.A.M.C. and the Q.A.I.M.N.S. Following the Great Retreat to the River Marne in 1914, the French Army medical service (*Service de Santé Militaire*) found itself stretched far beyond what it could handle. Desperate for nursing personnel, officials reached out across the Channel for help and the French Flag Nursing Corps (F.F.N.C.) was born, a collaborative effort between the French government, two prominent nurses in Britain — Mrs. Bedford Fenwick and Miss Grace Ellison — and their supportive committee. The British ladies were determined to recruit a steady supply of British (and, by extension, Canadian) nurses for French medical hospitals who would not only provide much-needed care, but also "raise the whole tone of nursing in France." In other words, they would rehabilitate the standards of French military nursing, which, by all British accounts, were adequate but cried for the precision, sanitation, and "cheeriness" that prevailed in British hospitals. Beginning in the latter half of 1914, approximately two hundred and fifty graduate nurses from Britain, Canada, Australia, and New Zealand who attested to being born of British parents and proficient in French signed up with the F.F.N.C., looking for a taste of the first aid experience behind French trenches. Because the French government expressly requested that no young women be sent, the minimum age was set at twenty-eight, later raised to thirty.

F.F.N.C. nurses typically worked in small groups of six or fewer, joining the staff of existing mobile hospitals near the firing line and stationary hospitals in the French interior. As nurses they accepted officers' rank in the French Army and until March 1917 the French government paid them a small salary and outfit allowance — so small as to make them nominal "volunteers." Travel and other expenses were to be paid out-of-pocket, and deficiencies in hospital supplies — such as gloves, thermometers, soap, and hot water bottles — were to be solicited from folks back home. Beginning in 1917, the British Branch (*Comité de Londres*) of the French Red Cross assumed financing and oversight responsibilities.

Evidently there were interpersonal obstacles to overcome in this arrangement. According to a contemporary (unabashedly pro-British) account, "Differences of custom and of religion...provide subtle opportunities for bruised feeling...But what may well cause wonder is that, with so many occasions of difficulty, things came to run so smoothly as on the whole they have done. The Sisters won their way to confidence by the excellence of their work." One can well imagine the tensions this situation suggested for nurses in the wards, and the journal *The Canadian Nurse* acknowledged that the linguistic, cultural, and practical challenges were "difficult for us, of course, but even more so for [the French]. Both contracting parties, however, have bravely stood the test, and have broken down all the barriers which might have proved insuperable."

Cool, brave heads were critical in the milieus of F.F.N.C. service. While some of its hospitals were permanent structures located well behind the front, many others took the form of *ambulances volants*, or "mobile ambulances." Not to be confused with motor ambulances, which were transport vehicles, these were rough barracks and tents erected close to the front, ready to be hastily dismantled and re-established as the army advanced or retreated. When the wind wasn't blowing the canvas down around their heads, nurses caught precious sleep in tiny bell tents while aircraft growled overhead and not-so-distant guns convulsed the ground. Night-duty nurses slept in broad daylight as convoys rumbled through and soldiers drilled just outside their tent flaps. "For a woman to be part of an ambulance like this is quite a new order of things," Grace Ellison wrote to her readership, for the F.F.N.C. promised acute danger and long hours at a time when the Canadian army had not yet introduced nursing sisters into its casualty clearing stations near the firing line. Recruitment appeals were fairly blunt about conditions: only women animated by a "pioneer spirit" need apply for this situation of discomfort and danger, surrounded by ruins and mud and sometimes lacking in basics such as four walls and someone to look after laundry. But, Ellison's letters urged, the satisfaction of lending desperately needed help to grateful *poilus*, the affectionate term in general use for the mustachioed and bearded French soldiers, was reward enough for the "true nurse." Indeed, F.F.N.C. nurses could boast of being in the vanguard — for example, they were among the first to occupy the devastated districts across the Hindenburg Line in 1918 — and many took home prestigious French military honours such as the *Croix de Guerre* and *Médaille des Épidémies*, awarded for persistent bravery under bombardment.

The scope of the F.F.N.C. sisters' mission differed in another major way from that of their Canadian military sisters: F.F.N.C. hospitals were less exclusively military and more available to the civil population. Whether or not the founders originally intended it that way, the F.F.N.C.'s mandate came to embrace whole villages, not just fighting men. F.F.N.C. work was as varied as it was relentless. In the absence of civilian doctors, F.F.N.C. nurses cared for local civilians, and fed and clothed refugees, often on their own time:

> We had a sad experience two nights about ten days ago
> when we were asked to meet two trainloads of refugees
> from the invaded districts...These poor, miserable people,
> so cold, hungry and travel-worn...all huddled up together
> in carriages without either light or warmth.... The snow
> lay thickly on the platform and it was bitterly cold. Being a
> very wretched night the Red Cross ladies were conspicuous
> by their absence, and we F.F.N.C. Sisters had the work
> to ourselves. This consisted in going from carriage to
> carriage with warm milk for the babies and small children,
> and plates of soup for the adults, with large chunks of
> war-bread....Poor things!...Our work being finished, we
> went off to our various abodes to snatch a few hours' sleep

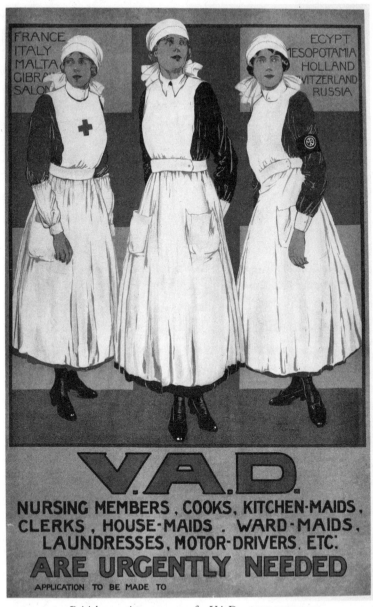

British recruitment poster for V.A.D.s. CWM 19920143-009

before getting-up time. On getting into my comfortable bed I thought of those tired homeless people spending such dreary hours on the hard train seats, after their trying dreadful experiences. The following night we were again told to meet a train of refugees.

On Christmas Day 1915, a contingent of ten Canadian nurses supervised by Miss Helen McMurrich, former instructor at Montreal General Hospital, sailed from Saint John, bound for the F.F.N.C. For their passage and equipment, they relied on the generosity of the Canadian public to the amount of $400 per nurse. During their stopover in England, they were invited into London's drawing rooms and theatres to catch an "idea of the greatness of London," all the while fortifying themselves with inspiration for their upcoming sacrifice. It was a breathless whirlwind of entertainments, sightseeing, and receptions that would stand in sharp contrast to next month's accommodations. By March, McMurrich and at least one other Canadian F.F.N.C. nurse were set up at Ambulance Mobile No. 1, a new surgical unit in the village of Rousbrugge, Belgium, and a gift of wealthy New Yorker Mary Borden Turner, herself a war nurse and author. Sister Agnes Warner had already been at this hospital for almost four months, looking forward eagerly to the extra pairs of Canadian hands that were rumoured to be on their way. She would soon praise them for being "a joy to work with, for they have had splendid training and are the kind that will go till they drop."

❧

Trained nurses were not the only ones intrigued by the prospect of high adventure and the pleasures of travel abroad. Thousands of other young, talented Canadian women longed to make a tangible contribution and see the world beyond their provincial neighbourhoods, but was there a role for them? Many could not produce a graduate certificate from an accredited nursing school, but had taken a St. John Ambulance course on basic nursing and were more than eager to learn on the job. In the face of the tens of thousands of young men who needed care, could not dogmatic insistence on formal training be set aside and non-nurses be allowed to serve for the duration? In Canada, the answer was a resounding "no": under no circumstances would the C.A.M.C. recruit untrained women for overseas nursing.

In taking this stance, Canadian authorities wanted to avoid the powder keg situation that had evolved in Britain with the pre-war formation of Voluntary Aid Detachments (V.A.D.s) — local groups of volunteer women recruited by the Red Cross and trained in brief courses by the St. John Ambulance to be called upon in an emergency. The more than 23,000 women who had joined Britain's V.A.D.s were a godsend in the crisis, but they also represented a threat to the status of trained nurses and a potential step back for the profession as a whole. If *any* woman could nurse, then training and certification would quickly become dispensable barriers to entry to the profession. Amateurs commanding lower rates of pay and privilege then might march into hospitals and set postwar nursing back to the nineteenth century.

And well-meaning "society ladies" who wanted to do their bit were actually getting in the way. On November 30, 1914, the Saint John *Daily Telegraph* reported the indignation of the profession when a hundred C.A.M.C. nurses crossed the Channel to take up their work at No. 1 Canadian General Hospital in Boulogne only to find that "lady amateurs [had] dispossessed them by buying their rooms over their head" for a higher rent. In Britain, where trained nurses were still struggling for protection through state registration, aristocratic women without any nursing experience were being allowed to assume positions of responsibility as directors or "lady superintendents" in war hospitals, a situation nurses chafed under and considered imminently dangerous to patients. *The British Journal of Nursing* regularly denounced "the inefficient amateur who, with practically no qualifications, is welcomed...smothered with lightly-earned brooches and medals, and given altogether false notions of her own value in national emergency." Editorialists among British nurses scorned the V.A.D.s as "undisciplined kittens," and dismissed their enthusiasm as "sentimental excitement" based on false ideas of what it meant to nurse.

They considered the V.A.D.s' quest for experience at the elbows of trained nurses a dangerous imposition. Occasionally, they lashed out with sarcasm at the higher-profile imposters: "[T]he half-penny papers have shown us some wonderful specimens of 'nurses in War dress'. . . . The Duchess of Westminster is quite in Puritan pose . . . with the addition of very high-heeled shoes and a liberal display of silk stocking. What the wonderful ruby and diamond cross suspended on her bosom denotes, we do not know, but the pet wolf-hound has gone along — and will, presumably, prevent its being snatched by the battle-field ghoul, when her Grace is under fire picking up the wounded." Other nurse editorialists were more admiring of the V.A.D.s' work and appreciative of their assistance, though still firmly critical of a system that continually betrayed trained nurses. Indeed, in Britain, the V.A.D. question was bound up with the wider struggle to elevate the nursing profession above that of domestic servant. British nurses, looking ahead, wanted to prevent thousands of volunteers swamping postwar hospitals claiming they had received their "training" in military wards and thus reducing the trained nurses' certificate to worthlessness.

Public opinion, though, failed to grasp the nuances of the debate, with many calling it "ungallant" to complain in time of crisis and the papers barely distinguishing between trained and untrained nurses. As far as onlookers on both sides of the Atlantic were concerned, anyone who signed up to help the wounded was to be commended — the privileged girl perhaps even more so for her greater sacrifice. Headlines such as "Society Girl Forsakes Social Frivols for Stern Duty of Nurse," published in a New Brunswick paper, rewarded and inspired similar acts of selflessness. Nonetheless, there was an undercurrent of suspicion that V.A.D.s might take advantage of their newfound freedoms abroad: a few postcards in circulation showed flirtations — or worse — between V.A.D.s and soldiers.

In Canada, a few thousand men and women were recruited as "V.A.D.s" early in the war to protect Canadians in various ways in the event of an invasion. The men were gradually absorbed by the army, but the women — mostly well-educated, unmarried, in their twenties and thirties, and middle class, who could afford both the training programs and the time for unpaid work — evolved into a volunteer nursing organization.

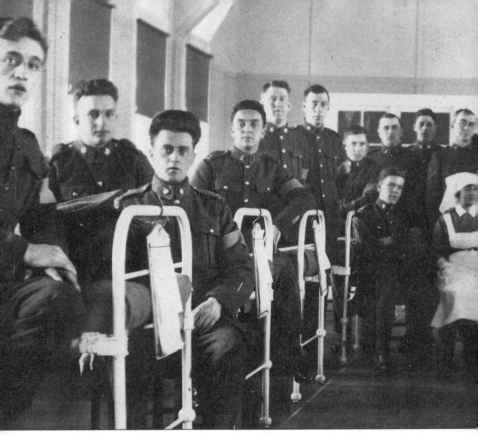

Convalescent ward at the New Brunswick Military Hospital in Fredericton.
NBM 1990.11.4

The Canadian military authorities took a practical view of V.A.D.s. The number of trained nurses who were applying to join the C.A.M.C. was sufficiently large that Canada did not have to turn to V.A.D.s to help fill the ranks. So, while V.A.D.s would not be permitted to work alongside the hospital and military-trained nurses of the C.A.M.C. — they lacked qualifications and the army could not vouch for their discipline — there might be a place for them as non-nursing assistants in military convalescent hospitals back in Canada, or as "home sisters" keeping house for trained nurses overseas in their billets or rest homes. Canadian V.A.D.s who wanted to nurse the wounded would still be welcomed by British

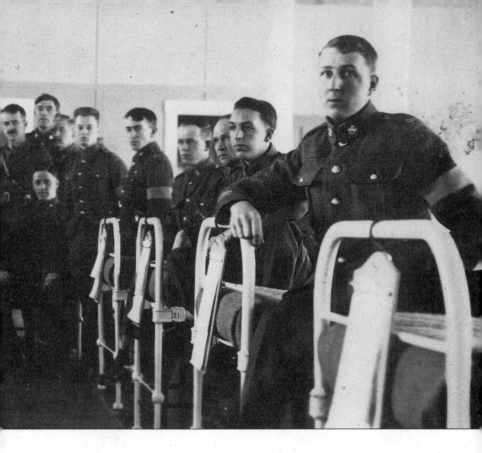

authorities, but only if they could get themselves across the Atlantic — and about five hundred did so.

From the beginning, then, a clear line in Canada indicated where serious, disciplined nursing ended and nursing "assistance" began. The line also struck through any aspirations women might hold of nursing full time without proper training. Consequently, Canada did not see the uglier side of the V.A.D. debate that was ongoing in Britain, although some of the young V.A.D.s who sailed for England from New Brunswick with local accolades ringing in their ears must have bumped abruptly into it

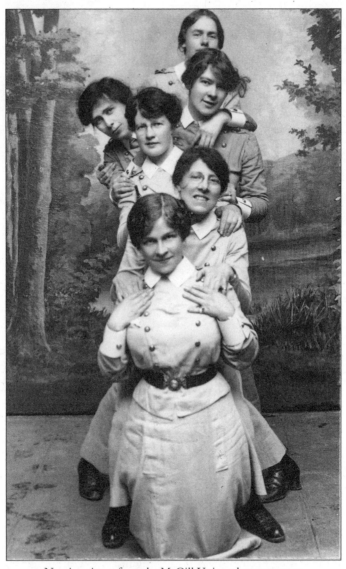

Nursing sisters from the McGill Unit on leave overseas.

NBM NANB-Military-7

on arrival. Fortunately, some hospitals managed to maintain a cooperative and friendly atmosphere between the nursing sisters and the V.A.D.s. And for the soldier-patients, who called them all "Sister," the differences in certification meant little or nothing.

As the war dragged on into its second year, there were nurses in blue, nurses in grey, nurses in white veils, nurses in black veils, volunteers with red crosses on their sleeves, and many variations in between. They bustled through the wards of giant general hospitals in England, lurched on hospital trains barrelling toward the French interior, slogged through inches of mobile ambulance mud, kept watch under dripping canvas marquees, shooed swarming flies from open wounds in the Mediterranean heat, or matured their sea legs on hospital ships plying the Atlantic. Though it might have been their second choice, some stayed home to nurse at convalescent soldiers' hospitals, where the need was also great. According to the *Daily Telegraph*, "up to October 5, 1916, the number of soldiers sent back to Canada because of medical unfitness was 6,208. Of these, 961 were suffering from wounds, shell-shock, or the effect of gas; 122 were insane; 245 were afflicted with tuberculosis; while the remainder, 4,880 were suffering from other diseases and disabilities." Those who needed artificial limbs or physical therapy to regain function had a long road ahead, and nurses were there to see them through their treatments.

While it is impossible to overstate how arduous were the challenges of nurses' on-duty hours, there were also hours of leisure and sheer exhilaration. Upon arrival in England, New Brunswick C.A.M.C. Sister Joyce Wishart and fellow nurses went on a grand tour of Buckingham Palace, the Tower of London, and the Guildhall. They visited an art gallery and took in a symphony concert at the Royal Albert Hall. In every direction lay a feast for the senses, mingled with corporeal reminders of a nation at war: "We don't hear much about the war, but you see soldiers everywhere, drilling in all the public squares and parks, while every taxi and wall is covered with patriotic appeals and mottoes, and the cry everywhere is for more men.... We have great fun here riding around on the high motor 'busses. They don't stop a second, but we go up and down the steps like squirrels." Soon the Canadian nurses settled into the hospital routine, whether in England or in France, but even then they were encouraged to make the most of their regular half-days, holidays, or leaves by enjoying the country they had come so far to see. Sister Clare Gass from Nova Scotia and her Miramichi friend Ruth Loggie purchased bicycles and raced around exploring the countryside of Boulogne and Étaples and seabathing on the French coast. To the vexation of British nursing authorities, Canadian nurses were even permitted to dance, provided it was with fellow officers at military events. With such a variety of edifying entertainments available to them, it was hoped Canadian nurses would not be tempted to break the rules and seek less legitimate forms of amusement, such as fraternization or intemperance, that might defame their service.

On the home front, family and citizens gobbled up nurses' letters and stories and tracked the comings and goings of local nurses. Saint John residents followed with special interest the vicissitudes of No. 1 Canadian General Hospital at Étaples, which was under the charge of Lieutenant-Colonel (Dr.) Murray MacLaren, who hailed from Saint John as did several of the nursing team. No. 2 Stationary Hospital at Le Touquet delighted newspaper readers in Canada by naming its wards after the provinces that had sponsored them.

The continued smooth operation of these hospitals was due at least in part to unflagging moral and material support from home. Women oversaw much of the fundraising through their local and provincial branches of the Red Cross, which organized the collection and sending not only of money, but also of supplies such as bandages, pillow slips, comfort bags (containing pencils, soap, candy, tobacco, and other useful items for soldiers), and bales of socks. Indeed, the emphasis on socks was quite remarkable, with periodic "sock drives" or "sock appeals" spurring knitters to new heights of production. Other philanthropic organizations participated, too, among them the Imperial Order Daughters of the Empire (I.O.D.E.), which collected socks as admission to its social events. Evidently, the sock drives succeeded, because thousands of warm pairs reached soldiers in time for winter, many with equally warm notes from New Brunswick ladies tucked into the toes. (Woe to the man who failed to remove the note before wearing!)

The Red Cross's policy was to supply the war zones as equitably as possible, rather than to deliver specific packages to particular hospitals on demand. Other philanthropic organizations, however, were free to post supply boxes directly to nurses who requested them, particularly those who worked for more loosely supported organizations such as the F.F.N.C. Individual chapters of the I.O.D.E., for instance, took charge of furnishing hospital supplies for individual nurses, as the De Monts chapter of the Saint John I.O.D.E. did for Sister Agnes Warner.

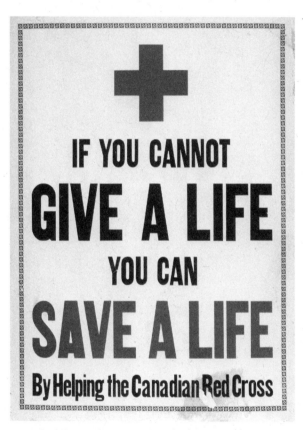

Red Cross poster appealing for financial support.
CWM 19900076-809

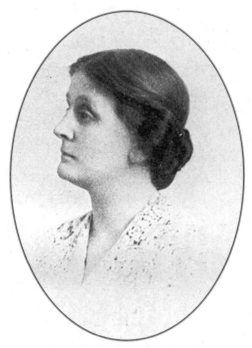

Agnes Warner. *My Beloved Poilus*

Chapter Three

Nursing Sister Agnes Warner

To say that Agnes Louise Warner was a New Brunswicker is only part of the truth. Born in 1872 to American parents living in Saint John, she maintained US citizenship and for several years trained and worked in New York City. But Saint John residents claimed the accomplishments of "the distinguished Saint John lady" as a source of great pride, and there is no doubt that "home" to Agnes was the city of her birth.

In her earliest years, the daughter of General Darius Bingham and Nancy Robinson Warner lived with older siblings Laura and John and younger siblings Richard, James, and Mary on the Rothesay Road overlooking Kennebecasis Bay. By about 1877, however, the family had moved, likely to the house they would continue to occupy well into the twentieth century, on the block bounded by Peel Street and Hazen Avenue. That year, five-year-old Agnes and her family mourned the death of Richard, just two, during a visit to Chicago. It was not the family's first tragic loss — a boy, Henry, had passed away at eight months in spring 1869 — but it was likely the first time little Agnes was forced to grapple with the frailty of human life and the permanence of loss.

In such a time, it probably helped Agnes to have remarkably resilient parents. Father Darius's illustrious military career during the Civil War had brought him steadily up through the ranks of the Union Army to brevet general, but cost him his arm in the Battle of Kennesaw Mountain. On his way to his new appointment as US consul in Saint John, the Ohio native married Nancy Robinson in Lancaster, Pennsylvania, and brought her to the New Brunswick harbour city, where he would endear himself against odds to a community initially apprehensive of Union military men. After serving as consul for twenty-two years, he went into the lumbering business with his brother and continued in active public life. The Warners remained based in Saint John, with continued ties and treks to Ohio, Illinois, and the Southern states throughout their lives.

Through her father, Agnes would have discovered a number of values that inspired her. Perhaps foremost among them was a sense of active citizenship and what it meant to take responsibility for one's fellow human beings in a crisis. In 1877, as a horrified citizenry surveyed the more than eighty smouldering hectares of the city core that had been swallowed by the Great Saint John Fire, General Warner "became the man of the hour." According to the *Saint John Globe,* he "telegraphed all over the US news of the calamity…and there was instantaneous and hearty response from many quarters." Warner set up an office at the local rink where the homeless were sheltering, and from this base assumed the duties of general superintendent overseeing the long-term relief committee and continuing to correspond with his contacts in the United States — notably Chicago — to establish a relief and recovery system.

This might be why the Warners were in Chicago when, just a few months after the fire, young son Richard died. Truly, it was a calamitous time for the family.

As she grew old enough to reflect on it, it must have struck Agnes how efficiently her father, by virtue of his military experience, had commanded the situation through the networks of contacts and organized supply he was able to set up. She saw his energy and people's confidence in his abilities despite the supposed debilitation of his missing arm. Years later, during a world war, Agnes would demonstrate the same qualities of coolness under pressure, resourcefulness in cultivating a network of supply, and, above all, a heartfelt responsibility for those tossed in the throes of crisis.

But first she would excel at home. Graduating with distinction from Victoria High School for Girls in 1890, she honed a natural interest in botany by participating in the province's Natural History Society (N.H.S.), no doubt encouraged by a leading botanist, George Upham Hay, who was principal at Victoria High, and by her own father, who sat on the society's executive. She studied local plants with interest, collected rare specimens, then skilfully dried, pressed, and labelled them for the N.H.S. — her specimens form part of the New Brunswick Museum's botanical collections to this day.

A few of her specimens came from Montreal, collected while she pursued an undergraduate degree at McGill University. In June 1893, the *Educational Review* reported that the third-year McGill student had achieved "second rank honors in natural sciences, first rank in general standing, honorable mention for collection of plants, and prize in mental philosophy." That summer Agnes stood up with her elder sister Laura ("Kit") as she married Saint John barrister Charles Coster in what the paper called the "society event of the season." Then it was back to McGill for a final banner year, which she finished off as a valedictorian of the Class of 1894.

Was it at this time that a future in nursing was brewing in Miss Warner's mind? With two grown daughters left at the Warner home, one could certainly be spared to travel, learn, and launch an independent career in a recently rehabilitated profession. By 1894, the number of reputable nursing schools had proliferated, leaving Agnes with many alternatives, including one at her doorstep: the Saint John General Hospital School for Nurses. But something made her pass on both this option and a second, obvious one: the new training program at the Montreal General Hospital.

Renowned nurse Anna Maxwell had established the Montreal school and briefly served as its superintendent in 1890 before moving on to found and direct the Presbyterian Hospital School of Nursing in New York City, and it was this latter institution that Warner chose to attend. Such a cross-border move was typical of her generation of New Brunswick women, many of whom left to find work or education in the New England states, and Agnes's US citizenship would have made the move that much easier. Indeed, from the absence of all but the Warner sons from the 1901 Saint John census, it is possible that much of her family joined her in the United States, which would not have been at all unusual for them, either. Agnes

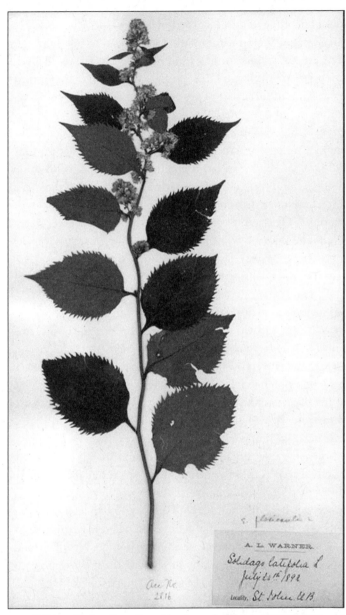

Solidago flexicaulis, collected by Agnes L. Warner. NBM VP-02816

might have had close friends or relatives in New York, but it was likely the reputation of the nursing school itself that attracted her, as it did others, such as Margaret Macdonald, future Matron-in-Chief of the C.A.M.C.

Whatever the particular appeal of New York and the Presbyterian Hospital School, Warner trained there, then remained as a private duty nurse for a wealthy couple on Long Island. It was common at the time for people of means to see their doctors at home and to hire private nurses to tend to their routine health care needs. A substantial fortune enabled Roswell and Louise Udall Eldridge to live an extravagant and somewhat cloistered lifestyle just outside the metropolis of New York. Warner became part of their extensive household, probably more like a member of the family than a servant, but still subject to the whims of the capricious Eldridges. (So intent on controlling their world were these two that, in 1911, they contrived to protect their estate from encroaching development and taxation by incorporating it as the Village of Saddle Rock, comprising servants and household members as taxpayers and voters, with themselves — first Mr., then Mrs. — as mayors.) The Eldridges had no children and they took frequent extended trips to Europe. This is how Agnes Warner came to be in France in August 1914, on the eve of the Great War.

It was probably not her first trip overseas with Mrs. Eldridge. This time the destination was Divonne-les-Bains, a village of about two thousand people on the Swiss border near Geneva that offered restorative spa accommodations in the shadow of the Alps. No doubt the party partook generously of the amenities at Divonne's Grand Hotel from the moment they arrived in May 1914. But that summer anyone with an ear to the ground would have detected the uneasy currents pulsing through the continent. Many locals reassured themselves that war might still be averted at the last moment, but on August 3 the church bells rang out all over France to herald the declaration, and Warner was there to witness it.

> On the very instant everyone knew what had happened.
> Gardeners, porters, all classes of men stopped work
> immediately and rushed to the city hall, where the same
> hour the proclamation of war was read and mobilization

started. The very next day 500 men of the village marched out in uniform — off to the front.... [M]any women, after preparing their husband's and their son's and brother's equipment, gave them all the money they possessed, thinking that they would need it to buy necessities. The same women were seen the next day working in various menial capacities to keep their families.

Two tense weeks passed during which restrictions on communications prevented any news of the war from reaching the village. In the meantime, there was no shortage of "thrilling incidents" to arouse fear and excitement. One of the hotel porters was discovered to be a spy reporting on the district to the enemy; the perpetrator managed to escape to Switzerland, but his complicit wife was imprisoned. A not-so-fortunate shoemaker in the town was found guilty and executed.

Within a few weeks, staff and volunteers had converted one wing of the Grand Hotel into a fifty-bed Red Cross hospital, though it was nearly a month before the wounded dispatched from the Alsace frontier would reach Divonne-les-Bains to convalesce. Warner was one of the first to volunteer for work in the makeshift hospital, even as most foreigners were fleeing the country for Switzerland. She also helped to train local women to provide basic nursing assistance.

When the wounded soldiers began to arrive, so did the more gruesome stories. But first the exhausted men had to sleep — one did so for thirty-five hours — and many slept so soundly that they had to be woken forcibly to eat. Others awoke after only a few minutes' rest, unaccustomed to the hush of the hospital after spending weeks assailed by the booming clamour of the battlefields — men who had finally learned to rest amid the roar of guns now could not sleep without it.

Stories of vicious enemy acts reached Warner through the soldiers and through her friend, Mme. Lalance, recently returned from Alsace, where she had operated a hospital for French soldiers. If previously Germans had been a faceless enemy in Warner's mind, a snarling, ruthless image quickly took shape through Mme. Lalance's reports. She heard how

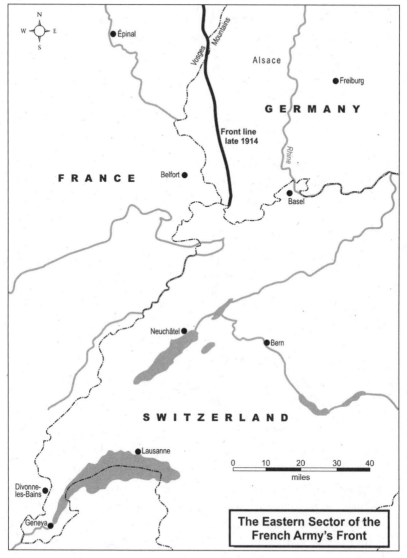

The Eastern Sector of the
French Army's Front

Mike Bechthold

German soldiers had stormed the hospital, held Lalance at the point of a pistol, ripped bandages from the bodies of the wounded to verify that they were truly impaired, and elsewhere shot a Red Cross nurse. Long before she got near the front, Warner's faith in the protection of the Red Cross symbol or in her chances of surviving an encounter with the enemy must have plummeted, replaced by a deeply buried but persistent fear that all her movements through the war zone were acutely dangerous.

But then, in mid-December, it was time to go home with Mrs. Eldridge. Christmas was right around the corner, and though the Eldridges generously supported the hotel-hospital at Divonne out of their pocketbooks, this was no place for a well-to-do American in tentative health. Warner would have to accompany them home, then snatch some much-needed holiday rest in Saint John. But images of penniless French women, their men gone to war, struggling to work their farms and feed their dependents; of worn-out, injured men; of need and want everywhere but "no grumbling" seized her with sympathetic admiration and the conviction that she would be "a coward and a deserter" if she did not share everything she had with these stoic people. Long before she left Divonne with the Eldridge household, Warner had resolved to get back to France.

She spent a few days in New York getting the Eldridges settled and arrived home in Saint John two days before Christmas. There was little time to rest, really, between talking to eager reporters about her activities, getting her passports in order, making her rounds among friends and family, and drumming up material support before her departure on January 13. This time she packed heavy, "taking with her quite a large supply of useful articles contributed by St. John friends who know the value of the work she is doing and the necessity for contributions," reported the *Daily Telegraph*. During her whirlwind mission, she must have encountered some confusion when she told people that, no, she was not nursing Canadian or British wounded, and, no, she was not working in a Canadian or British hospital, for the *Daily Telegraph* went on to note that

> Miss Warner feels that our people do not sufficiently
> recognize the magnificent courage and spirit of sacrifice

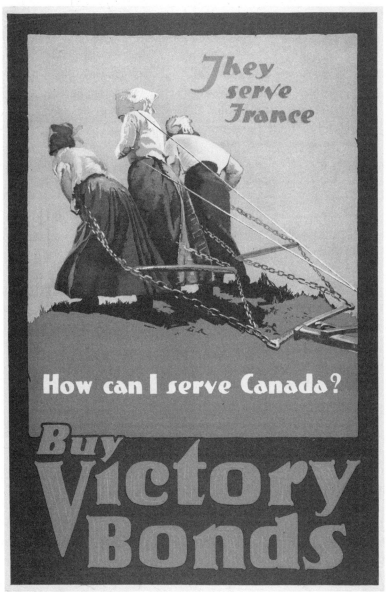

Canadian Victory Bonds poster using the example of French women to encourage Canadians. McGill University WP1.B12.F2

shown by the French people. She reminds her friends, in talking, of these things, that while the British have done heroic work, the greater part of the long line from the Belgian coast across to Switzerland, a curving line of 200 miles, is defended by the French. The whole French nation, men, women and children, she says, are deserving of the gratitude and admiration of the world.

Evidently Warner's plea was persuasive: not only did her baggage bulge with supplies, but for the next four years a steady stream of packages and cash from her native Saint John would flow unabated.

Back on French soil, Warner spent an eye-opening few weeks at the American Ambulance in Paris, observing exciting surgical innovations that encouraged her. But soon she felt beckoned by the need at Divonne-les-Bains. As an American "neutral" not contracted to any organization in particular, Warner was free to move autonomously. With nothing urgent to keep her in Paris, she returned to Divonne in February 1915 to be welcomed back as the darling of the village.

As before, her practise of care in Divonne extended well beyond the hospital into the homes of soldiers' families. For a war nurse, it was a unique, discretionary mission: at a time when her military counterparts focused most of their efforts on hospital work, Warner cast a wider net. Wherever she was posted, she drew deeply from her (informal) channels of trans-Atlantic supply to find comfort items and money for the most destitute families in the area. She also found ways to stretch and multiply the Saint John donations with schemes that enabled European women and children to supply goods for the insatiable war. When every society in Saint John was busy collecting socks for soldiers, Warner asked her friends to collect yarn, too, which she turned over to village women to knit into socks, thereby offering them the dual advantage of outfitting their fighting men *and* earning a small income for their families. Her continual shopping, soliciting, saving, and hoarding soon earned her the reputation of a packrat — good naturedly, of course, because anyone could see how quickly these precious articles passed through her hands to those who needed them most. That she even found the time to organize and allocate them while working long hours in the wards suggests an extraordinary efficiency on Warner's part. It also demonstrates how clearly she understood that easing an anxious soldier's mind about the condition of loved ones back home made it easier for him to keep on with the grim work of recovery — just as a cheery word about his recovery could shore up the spirits of his toiling family.

In April, officials began talking about expanding the hospital to four hundred beds and putting it under military control, with Warner in charge of nursing. No doubt she was the most senior nurse currently at the hospital, and this impressive promotion would have seemed natural to the authorities. But Warner's first thought was one of reluctance to take on the daunting red tape of military bureaucracy. Perhaps as an attempt to educate herself on the administration of larger operations, that May she took a brief tour of hospitals in the Lyon area. After returning, she took charge of at least a sizeable portion of the Divonne hospital and remained there for the summer. But she had another field in mind.

That September, Warner suddenly announced that she was thrilled to be moving to an ambulance close to the front, where she would have "a chance to do good work" and be "nearer the Canadian boys." This was an incentive she shared with many other nurses: all longed to work where there was the greatest need and the greatest chance of seeing familiar faces. Though she knew little about it before arriving, her next post would be with the F.F.N.C. at Mary Borden Turner's newly established Ambulance Mobile No. 1 in Rousbrugge, Belgium, only twenty kilometres from the strategically important and oft-assailed city of Ypres, and within sixteen kilometres of the front — so close that the wounded could reach her operating room before infection set in.

Turner may have known of Warner prior to 1915, and they certainly had been in touch earlier that year. Whatever the nature of their prior acquaintance, from early on Warner clearly had the trust and respect of "Mrs. Turner," herself a Red Cross nurse (though not a trained one) serving as *la directrice* of the ambulance she had founded. It is interesting to speculate about the relationship between these two women, particularly in

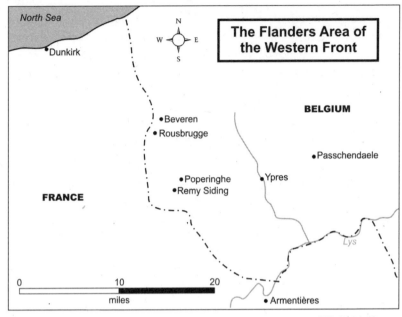

Mike Béchthold

light of Turner's postwar publication, *The Forbidden Zone,* a probing literary reflection on her experience during the war. In a frank and controversial work that dispenses with the romantic veneer of wartime nursing narratives, Turner confronts the moral contradictions of nursing men's bodies only to send them back to be re-abused, and she challenges assumptions about what was appropriate for women writers to articulate about suffering. From Warner's brief remarks about their interactions and from Warner's rapid elevation to *infirmière major* (matron) in charge of the ambulance, it is clear that the two women worked closely together in mutual trust. In the stolen moments of conversation, did they disclose a kindred sensibility; did they share a thoughtful critique of the way their grim world was being managed? Whatever they discussed, the postwar world would neither read a frank appraisal from Agnes Warner, who never published one, nor readily welcome Mary Borden Turner's perspective.

Many of the other trained nurses in Ambulance Mobile No. 1 at

Rousbrugge were F.F.N.C. nurses — hailing from the British Empire and the United States — who worked outside the British military system, moving instead with the French army, with teams of French doctors, caring largely for French *poilus*, and receiving French military decorations for their most gallant acts. To Warner's delight, many of the nurses in the area were Canadian. Helen McMurrich, supervisor of the first Canadian unit of nurses to join the F.F.N.C., arrived in Rousbrugge in March 1916 and quickly hit it off with Warner. They travelled together when they went on leave and were still working together well into 1919. Not far away, in Rémy Siding, near Poperinghe, Saint John Nursing Sister Margaret Hare had charge of the busy No. 3 C.C.S. Warner visited her from time to time to compare notes, help with dressings, or observe surgeries. Best of all was the promise that her beloved nephew "B" (Robert Warner Bayard Coster) might be discovered somewhere near the front — indeed, he turned up in a camp near Ypres after some diligent reconnaissance on the part of his Aunt Warner.

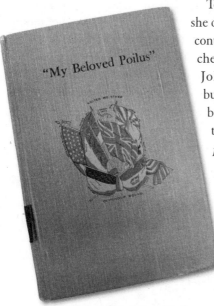

Cover of *My Beloved Poilus*.

To add to the Canadian camaraderie she discovered in her new post, Warner continued to receive care packages and cheques addressed to her from Saint John. While she was now much busier with urgent cases than she had been in Divonne, she still scrambled to distribute articles and cash to her *poilus* and their families. There is little doubt that chapter members Mary Warner and Laura (Warner) Coster had something to do with keeping their sister Agnes's efforts in the hearts and minds of the De Monts chapter of the I.O.D.E., which continued to donate prodigiously. Supply shortages were a fact of life at hospitals such as Mobile No. 1 — as Nurse Warner continually reminded her supporters, it was thanks to their generosity that she was able to help as many soldiers as she did.

Then someone had an idea to amplify her message. Without actually consulting Warner, a group of friends gathered excerpts from her 1914-1916 letters to Saint John family and friends and contracted local printers Barnes and Co. to publish them in book form. By March 1917, local businesses were selling copies of *My Beloved Poilus* for $1.00 each, and proceeds from the little chronicle began reaching Warner herself shortly thereafter. What must she have thought about this well-intentioned parade of her private letters before a much broader audience? Did she know that even former premier (and soon-to-be lieutenant governor) William Pugsley was presenting copies as "souvenirs" to the dozens of V.I.P.s he entertained? It is unlikely that she worried about the content of *My Beloved Poilus* — skulky friends still can make trustworthy editors. The published letters had been modified and condensed with discretion, and none of her more intimate notes, if she wrote any, was allowed to stray into *My Beloved Poilus*. But she was uneasy about the unpolished style of her letters. To her mother she confided, "I must say it was an awful shock when I first received it, but if the people are interested, in spite of the appalling English, and it sells well, I must not mind. You know I did not even have time to read over my letters and they are rather a disgrace to a graduate of McGill."

In throwing back the tent flap and giving the reader a glimpse of the daily rhythms of hospital life, the letters of *My Beloved Poilus* are illuminating, but inevitably limited by the nature of wartime correspondence. Long before the Saint John "editors" took their turn, Warner herself would have filtered the details to obscure the location and movements of her hospital to satisfy the military censors. This caution is much more pronounced in her letters from the Belgian front than in those written farther back at Divonne-les-Bains, and the need for it must have frustrated correspondents on both sides of the Atlantic. The nurses themselves, however, typically were kept in the dark about the army's movements and could only speculate (from patterns of gunfire and numbers of wounded) about what was going on around them. In such conditions, rumours thrived and anxieties simmered as nurses waited for real news.

Quite apart from the dictates of censorship, nurses had other reasons to check their tone and convey a strategic impression when writing letters. Motives were as much personal as political, for if a nurse was unable to remain duly selfless and optimistic — even "cheerful" — about her part in restoring the wounded to victory, where would that leave her or her dependent charges and the possibility of re-establishing life as she once knew it? Despondency and introspection were dangerous when everything depended on swift and passionate action; a "chin-up" attitude was crucial for encouraging sustained contributions of men, materiel, and morale from home. Figuring prominently in Sister Warner's letters, therefore, are the ongoing needs of the soldiers, the hardships borne bravely by local women, the triumphs of recovery, and gratitude for contributions. Her tone, though, is practical and matter-of-fact, rather than probingly reflective. In any case, clutching the stub of a pencil in her frozen fingers after eighteen hours on her feet, she did not have *time* to ruminate on what she had experienced, let alone wax literary. But she would summon her most earnest eloquence in detailing for bereaved French families the last brave hours their men had spent in her hospital before succumbing to their wounds. Then she might have a few minutes to scribble a letter home — lighter fare, though no less obligatory, even though there must have been moments when Warner was sorely tempted to bypass pen and paper for the relative rapture of just closing her eyes and ending the day.

As a trained nurse, Warner was no stranger to the gruesome sight and heavy smell of infection, the sickening cross-section of severed limbs, or the unnerving actions of a dying man. The gleaming blades and points of hospital instruments, the bustle of routine, the pressures of assisting at operations, the position one adopted when leaning over a miserable patient — all had long since been part of her reality but not subjects about which to write home. But now she was forced to come to grips with horror writ large: families torn apart, women struggling to feed their families, convoys of refugees, muddy, shattered soldiers. All this, combined with

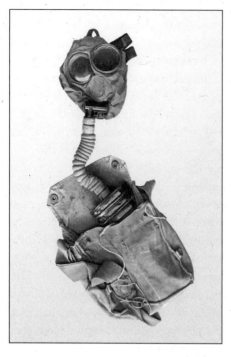

British gas mask known
as a Small Box Respirator.
CWM 19720102-061

the perennial shortage of materials and personnel to meet the need, would have presented impossibilities she had never encountered at the New York Presbyterian Hospital School for Nurses. The need to heal the desperately wounded, moreover, was leading to new techniques, such as "plastic" surgery to reconstruct demolished faces, therapeutic massage, and new methods of dressing gangrenous wounds to permit ongoing irrigation with a germicidal treatment known as Dakin's (or Carrel-Dakin) solution. Dakin's treatment posed a special challenge for nurses because it required almost constant adjustment to manage the tubes and pumps — but it reduced the rate of amputations, which nurses were eager to avoid.

But new healing techniques could not keep pace with the sinister inventions of wartime: guns that hurled shells faster, farther; aircraft that dropped death and dismemberment from the sky; and, perhaps worst of all, vicious poison gases that swept into Allied trenches and choked all hope of recovery for thousands. Causing debilitating chemical burns on the skin and respiratory membranes of the patient, contamination with chlorine, phosgene, and, later, "mustard" gas could easily claim a man's life — or worse (Warner felt), his eyesight. The pain of gas burns was often unendurable and the nursing arduous. Some cases had to be protected by bed tents against contact of any kind except careful swabbing with neutralizing solutions. Warner first mentions gas on her arrival at the front in September 1915, when both sides were using chlorine and phosgene weapons. In 1916, she declared gas "the worst thing I have seen yet" — not a superlative to be taken lightly from a nurse who had treated every variant of hideousness the war had manufactured to date. (Mustard gas, introduced by the Germans in 1917, had even grislier effects.) Despite the foul smell of gas masks and the inconvenience of working in them, nurses must have been grateful to have them.

Apart from gingerly handling gas casualties and dressing shell wounds, nurses also tended to men suffering from epidemic illnesses (pneumonia, dysentery, and trench fever), many which were spread through contact with decaying flesh, vermin, and filth in the trenches. Such cases occupied a certain percentage of beds in any war hospital: the "ill, not wounded." Nurses near the front came in contact with their share of decaying flesh, swarming rats, lice, and filth, too, and they struggled to keep their areas, aprons, and starched cuffs clean. Special precautions, such as rubber gloves, kerosene shampoos, and meticulous grooming were essential to prevent septic fingers and infections. Cold, wet winters added to the burden, as long-term exposure to the elements left many soldiers (and occasionally nurses) with crippling rheumatism or frostbite.

Some ailments, despite their prevalence among the soldiers, are mentioned only rarely in contemporary accounts. One was nerve strain (alternately, "nerve paralysis" or "shell shock"), a condition that included disorientation, localized paralysis, mutism, or muscle tics brought on by psychological reactions to horrific experiences at the front. Early in the war medical personnel tended to consider it temporary insanity or emotional collapse — something that would melt away in a restorative setting such as Divonne-les-Bains. But the rising number of disabling cases represented a serious threat to manpower and prompted military authorities to become serious about getting victims back in fighting condition as soon as possible. The typical prescription — segregation and therapy at the hands of an exacting medical team — was not calibrated to be sympathetic, but to "re-educate the will" through exposure to demanding situations, discipline, and sometimes electric shock applied to uncooperative parts of the body. Whether the shocks were intended to be strictly therapeutic, partly motivational, or largely punitive is not clear, and may have depended on the administrator. It is evident from Warner's letters that the hospital in Divonne-les-Bains offered electrical treatment. Though she only identifies its recipients as "paralyzed," rather than "nerve paralyzed" or "insane," the fact that so many of them reportedly regained their mobility under treatment suggests they may have suffered from shell shock.

The other hushed condition was venereal disease, sufferers of which typically were removed to separate hospitals or treated by male orderlies rather than by female nurses.

❖❖

As 1915 gave way to a new year of fighting, the bombardments grew so severe that the numbers and condition of the wounded pouring into Mrs. Turner's ambulance at times overwhelmed the staff. The wards were so full that when a wounded General Lerous arrived, nurses struggled to find the mandatory space to segregate him from the rank-and-file wounded, and furthermore to accommodate his wife and the Belgian royalty who came to visit him. (Royal visits to hospitals were relatively common events during the war; besides cheering the soldiers, they served to buoy the spirits of the staff and boost their visibility with war authorities and sponsors — Warner's hospital was no exception.)

Unfortunately for Warner, the frantic pace that spring meant she had to postpone the rest trip to Divonne she had planned for March. When she finally was able to leave the roar of the front in May, her first sleep was as long as it was restful. But just like the soldiers she used to receive at the Divonne hospital, the next night she found it too quiet to sleep.

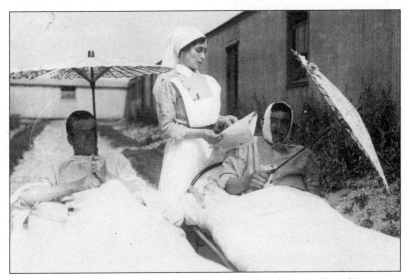

C.A.M.C. nurse at a hospital reads the news from home to Canadian convalescents. CWM 19920085-529

Presumably, as a requisite to service in the F.F.N.C., Warner was proficient in French, thanks in part to her Victorian education and the time she spent in Montreal. Proficiency would have been critical for managing good relationships with doctors, orderlies, and patients alike, and Sister Warner seems to have been singularly successful (or fortunate) in forging harmony with all three. Her letters are free of the exasperation shown in other nurses' accounts toward the untrained help, possibly because her orderlies (and also the "nurses," or "*infirmiers*" as she tended to refer to them, notwithstanding that they were amateur) were motivated French citizens rather than the P.O.W.s or "inept soldier" orderlies of British and Canadian military hospitals, who required close, prodding supervision. It is also likely that she commanded respect through her leadership abilities and attracted local affection with her relief work beyond the hospital. The humility in her letters certainly suggests that, after taking charge as matron in 1916, Warner led her colleagues by earnest example. In contrast with the matrons of larger military hospitals whose chief duties were oversight and discipline, she obviously participated fully as a ward nurse alongside her close-knit staff. It is noteworthy that, in so many of her sentences composed in Belgium, the subject is "we."

Faced with mind-numbing toil and pain, nurses did whatever they could to lighten things up for themselves and the men. They planned and hosted entertainments, usually located on site so patients could participate. They lavishly summoned Christmas in the wards with festoons, songs, and treats — clearly a lot of work but unquestionably worth the trouble. No one viewed decorations as frivolous in a wartime hospital; rather, colourful ribbons, flowers, and blankets were an integral part of the restorative therapy nurses designed for patients — part of that tidy, heavenly atmosphere soldiers ascribed to the nurses' sovereignty in the wards. Even a poorly heated barrack ward was nothing less than a palace next to the shivering, swarming miseries of grey trench life.

In truth, nurses embroidered their world as much for their own sake as for their patients'. An endless visual diet of grey walls, white sheets, brown mud, and red wounds had the effect of super-sensitizing the retina to colour and beauty, causing nurses to linger in doorways, enchanted by sunrises over the Belgian countryside, and to hover over flower arrangements picked by recovering patients eager to show their gratitude. We know that Warner had a zeal for plants from an early age, and it finds expression in her *My Beloved Poilus* letters. But in those surroundings, it becomes more spiritual than academic — like many nurses who sprinkle their accounts with glimpses of beauty, she interprets that beauty as Hope.

Personal joy might have been rare in the frenzied nights and days, but it would not have taken much to liberate a laugh from a human spirit craving mirth. A kitten's brazen antics, a friendly message dropped by an air force pilot, or a patient's quip could easily coax a smile from a nurse, and everyone was eager to earn one. If we are to believe the claim of Warner and other nurses that their soldier-patients were nothing if not perfect gentlemen — or, rather, "boys" — then it seems to have been relatively uncomplicated for nurses to maintain an easy, familial rapport. As long as men viewed nurses as religious or domestic "Sisters" and nurses considered themselves stand-in mothers to grateful children, all could enjoy a respectfully affectionate relationship in which nurses showed warmth without compromising professionalism. More likely, there were occasional lapses of patience or decorum on the part of both parties in an atmosphere of disgust, desire, madness, pain, and long-term deprivation. But reports of unseemly behaviour rarely made it across the Atlantic. On the contrary, nurses praised the manners and restraint of the soldiers and even indulged in national comparisons of their pluck:

> At one hospital where nearly all the patients were French, several Canadians were brought in, among them a brawny chap named McDonald. The Poilus were very curious to see how this Canadian would behave, and as he had a bad dressing to be done Miss Warner was anxious that he should be as brave as the French. However, she saw his face getting red, and she said to him, 'Well, if it will make you feel better, say it.' And the Canadian opened his mouth and ejaculated, 'Boys!' The Colonel of his regiment, who came to the hospital later, told Sister Warner that McDonald could do better than that, as he was a foreman of the railway construction line and had quite a command of the language.

Another good reason to behave oneself in front of the nurse was the discretion she wielded. A good word from her to the medical officer might prolong a soldier's convalescence period and keep him off the "fit for duty" list awhile longer — possibly even send him home.

❧

What Sister Warner's eager New Brunswick readership got in *My Beloved Poilus* was a series of snapshots — both visual and narrative — of her adopted world. Amid the unrelenting rhythms of work and care, she highlights her own experience of uncertainty, discomfort, joy, and revulsion. We get to know how strongly she feels about senseless devastation and how heavily she relies on support from home. We see how keeping busy sustains her mentally and how the *poilus'* gratitude restores her emotionally. In the letters are glimpses of her inner struggle to sort out her feelings on the war's lethal perplexities — wondering how to reconcile her fear and her pride when nephew Bayard signs up as a soldier or rethinking her position on nursing the enemy when German soldiers first arrive in her hospital in May 1916. And despite a momentary vow to give up nursing altogether after the war, we see her taking every opportunity to augment her professional knowledge of surgical advancements and methods of hospital administration by touring other facilities. Through the letters, we move ever closer to the front lines with a dedicated woman who takes one difficult day at a time.

As she was writing the last letter that would be bound into *My Beloved Poilus*, neither Warner nor her readers could have contemplated that her ordeal at the front was scarcely more than half over.

Chapter Four

My Beloved Poilus

Preface

When Florence Nightingale began her great work in
the hospital wards at Scutari in 1854,[1] she little realised
how far-reaching would be the effect of her noble
self-sacrificing efforts. Could she today visit the war-
stricken countries of Europe she would be astonished
at the great developments of the work of caring for the
wounded soldiers which she inaugurated so long ago.
Her fine example is being emulated today by hundreds of
thousands of brave women who are devoting themselves
to the wounded, the sick, and the dying in countless
hospital wards.

All too little is known of what these devoted nurses
have done and are doing. Some day the whole story will
be given to the world; and the hearts of all will be thrilled
by stirring deeds of love and bravery. In the meantime it
is pleasing and comforting to catch fleeting glimpses of
a portion of the work as depicted in this sheaf of letters,

---

[1] Nurse Florence Nightingale and her staff worked in a hospital in Scutari, Turkey,
caring for wounded and sick British soldiers during the Crimean War.

now issued under the title of *My Beloved Poilus*, written from the front by a brave Canadian nurse.

Two outstanding features give special merit to these letters. They were not written for publication, but for an intimate circle of relatives and friends. And because of this they are not artificial, but are free and graceful, with homely touches here and there which add so much to their value. Amidst the incessant roar of mighty guns; surrounded by the wounded and the dying; shivering at times with cold, and wearied almost to the point of exhaustion, these letters were hurriedly penned. No time had she for finely turned phrases. Neither were they necessary. The simple statements appeal more to the heart than most eloquent words.

These letters will bring great comfort to many who have loved ones at the front. They will tell them something of the careful sympathetic treatment the wounded receive. The glimpses given here and there, of the efforts made by surgeons and nurses alike to administer relief, and as far as possible to assuage the suffering of the wounded, should prove most comforting. What efforts are made to cheer the patients, and to brighten their lot, and what personal interest is taken in their welfare, are incidentally revealed in these letters. For instance, "The men had a wonderful Christmas Day (1916). They were like a happy lot of children. We decorated the ward with flags, holly, and mistletoe, and paper flowers that the men made, and a tree in each ward."

How these letters bring home to us the terrible tragedy that is going on far across the ocean. And yet mingled with the feeling of sadness is the spirit of inspiration which comes from the thought of those brave men who are offering themselves to maintain the right, and the

devoted women who are ministering to their needs.
Our heads bow with reverence, and our hearts thrill with
pride, when we think of them. But we must do more than
think and feel; we must do our part in supporting them
and upholding their hands. They have given their all.
They can do no more, and dare we do less?

Rev. H.A. Cody
Saint John, N.B.
February 19, 1917

Introduction

The writer of these letters, a graduate of McGill College,
and the Presbyterian Hospital, New York, left New York
in the spring of 1914 with a patient for the continent
finally locating at Divonne-les-Bains, France, near the
Swiss border, where they were on August 1, when war
broke out. She immediately began giving her assistance
in Red Cross work, continuing same until the latter part
of November, when she returned with her patient to
New York — made a hurried visit to her home in Saint
John, and after Christmas returned to again take up the
work which these letters describe.

My Beloved Poilus

August 2, 1914
Divonne-les-Bains, France

Dear Mother:

The awful war we have all been dreading is upon us — *France Is Mobilizing*. At five o'clock yesterday morning the tocsin sounded from the *Marie* (village hall) and men, women, and children all flocked to hear the proclamation which the Mayor of the village read. It called upon all of military age — between twenty years and fifty years — to march at once, and inside of twenty-four hours five hundred men had gone, they knew not where. The bravery of these villagers — men and women — is remarkable, and not to be forgotten. No murmuring, no complaining — just, *ma patrie*, tying up the little bundle — so little — and going; none left but old men, women, and children.

We have started teaching the women and girls to make bandages, sponges, etc., for the hospital which will be needed here.

August 23, 1914
Divonne-les-Bains, France

Your letter came yesterday — twenty days on the way — but I was fortunate to get it at all; so many of these poor people, whose nearest and dearest have gone to fight for their country, have had no word from them since they marched away, and they do not know where they are.

From this little village five hundred men left the first day of mobilization; there is not a family who has not some one gone, and from some both fathers and sons have gone, as the age limit is from twenty to fifty years.

I am filled with admiration and respect for these people. The courage of both the men and women is remarkable. There is no hesitation, and no grumbling, and everyone tries to do whatever he or she can to help the cause.

I do not know if I told you, in my last letter, of the poor lady who walked all night through the dark and storm to see her son who was leaving the next morning. All the horses and motors had been taken by the government for the army, so she started at eleven o'clock at night, all by her self, and got here about five in the morning — her son left at seven, so she had two hours with him. While there are such mothers in France she cannot fall. There are many such stories I might tell you, but I have not the time.

The Red Cross has started a branch hospital here, and I have been helping them to get it in order. It is just about ready now, and we may get soldiers any day.

I have classes every morning and find many of the women very quick to learn the rudiments of nursing. Every one in the place is making supplies and our sitting room is a sort of depot where they come for work.

If my patient is as well in October as she is now I am going to stay and give my services to the Red Cross. If I have to go home with her I will come back — I would be a coward and deserter if I did not do all I could for these poor brave people.

October 25, 1914

Another Sunday — but this is cold and rainy — the days slip by so quickly I cannot keep track of them. We have only two soldiers left at the hospital — they tell us every day that others are coming. The country all about is perfectly beautiful with the autumn coloring. We do not see any of the horrors of the war here. If it were not for the tales that come to us from outside, and for the poor broken men who come back, we would not know it was going on. There are very enthusiastic accounts of the Canadians in all the English papers.

About February 15, 1915
Paris

Back safely in Paris after taking my patient to New York and a short visit home, which now seems like a dream.

I have been spending a lot of time at the American Ambulance this week, but have not gone out to stay as yet, as I still have to see some other small hospitals and had to go to the clearing house to make arrangements for sending supplies, which I brought from home and New York, to different places.

I have seen quite a number of operations, and as X-ray pictures are taken of all the cases there is no time wasted in hunting for a bullet; they get the bullet out in about two minutes. They are using Dr. Criles' anaesthetic — nitrous oxide gas and oxygen — it has no bad effects whatever. The patients come out of it at once as soon as the mask is taken off, and there is no nausea or illness at all; and most of them go off laughing, for they cannot believe that it is all over — they feel so well; but oh, mother, it is awful to see the sad things that have happened. In some cases there are only pieces of men left. One young chap, twenty-one years old, has lost both legs. At first he did not want to live, but now he is beginning to take an interest in things and is being fitted for wooden legs.

The dental department have done wonderful work. They build up the frame work of the face and jaws, and then the surgeons finish the work by making new noses and lips and eyelids. I thought I had seen a good many wonderful things, but I did not believe it possible to make anything human out of some of the pieces of faces that were left, and in some of the cases they even get rid of the scars. Photos are taken when they first come in, and then in the various stages of recovery. One of the worst cases I saw the last day I was out. He has to have one more operation to fill in a small hole in one side of his nose and then he will be all right.

Last Sunday one of the men in Miss B___'s ward was given the medal for distinguished service. He had saved his officer's life — went right out before the guns and carried him in on his back. He was struck himself just before he got to his own lines and one leg almost torn off. When they brought him

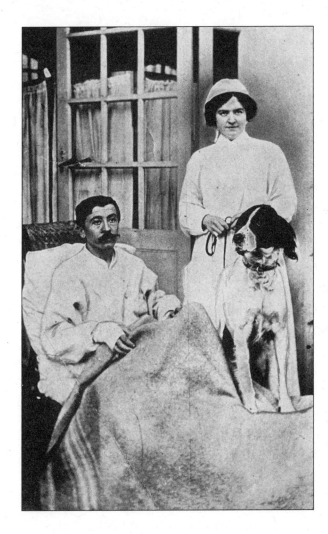

The dog who saved his master's life. *My Beloved Poilus*

to the American Ambulance, all the doctors, except Dr. B____, said his leg would have to come off at once — he refused to do it and saved the leg for the man. It will be stiff, of course, as the knee joint is gone entirely; but will be better than a wooden leg, and the poor man is so pleased.

I must tell you about the wonderful dog that is at the American Ambulance; perhaps you have read about him in some of the papers. His master came from Algeria, and of course did not expect to take his dog with him, but when the ship left the wharf the dog jumped into the sea and swam after it, so they put off a boat and hauled him on board, and he has been with his master all through the war. He was in the trenches with him, and one day a German shell burst in the trench and killed all of his companions and buried this man in the mud and dirt as well as injuring him terribly. Strange to say the dog was not hurt at all, and the first thing the man remembered was the dog digging the mud off his face. As soon as he realized his master was alive he ran off for help, and when they were brought into the ambulance together there were not many dry eyes about. After he was sure his master was being taken care of he consented to go and be fed, and now he is having the time of his life. He is the most important person in the place. He has a beautiful new collar and medal, lives in the diet kitchen, and is taken out to walk by the nurses, and best of all is allowed to see his master every day. I will send a photo of him to you. His master has lost one leg, the other is terribly crushed, and one hand also, but Dr. B____ thinks he can save them.

I think I shall go back to Divonne-les-Bains — they are urging me so strongly and there seems to be more need there.

February 19, 1915

Back again in Divonne-les-Bains. It seems as if I had never been away — I have fallen into the old work so easily. I left Paris Sunday night about eight o'clock and arrived here at two the next day, and had a warm welcome from everybody. One poor man died of tetanus before I got back. I have nine on my floor. I have thirteen patients, nine in bed all the time, and the others up part of the day. One of the women of the village helps me in the morning, two others help with the cleaning up and serving meals; everything has to be carried up three flights of stairs, so you can imagine the work.

I have a very comfortable room at the hotel, go to the ambulance at seven in the morning and generally get back at nine or half past. I do not know how long I shall be here — until this lot get well or more come.

One of the patients is a chef, and was acting as cook for the regiment when a shell landed in his soup pot; he was not wounded, but his heart was knocked out of place by the shock and his back was twisted when he fell.

February 28, 1915

The poor man who was so very ill died on the morning of the twenty-third after three weeks of intense suffering — I stayed that night with him. The others are all out of danger with the exception of two who cannot get well — one is paralyzed and the other has tuberculosis.

I went to the village for the first time yesterday and was quite touched by the welcome I received at every little shop and house. The people seemed genuinely glad to have me back. They cannot seem to get over the fact that I have crossed the ocean twice and come back to them. To them the ocean is a thing of terror, especially since the war broke out. Dr. R____ has a great many sick people in the country about here to take care of in addition to the soldiers. In one house they had nothing to eat but potatoes, but he is a good deal like our dear old doctor, and feeds and clothes and takes care of them himself.

March 5, 1915

I can scarcely believe that it is nearly three weeks since I left Paris. I have been so busy, that the days fly by. Some of the men are leaving tomorrow, and most of the others are getting along very well.

Mr. E____ [possibly Mr. Eldridge, her patient's husband] is indeed kind. He has just sent an order to the village people, who make beautiful lace and embroidery, for $500 worth of work. They are so happy about it, for it means food for many of them. One poor woman, who has lost her husband in the war and has a child to take care of, can earn only eighteen francs a month, that is $3.60, and that is all she has to live on.

March 7, 1915

One of the American doctors from the American Ambulance came to see me yesterday. He was very much interested in what he saw and is coming back in ten days. We have had one or two beautiful days, the pussy-willows are beginning to come out, and primroses everywhere.

Dr. S___ said that the man who owned the wonderful dog that is at the American Ambulance is really getting well, and they managed to save one leg and the crushed hand.

In Dr. B___'s service he did not do a single amputation during the months of January and February — a very wonderful record.

Dr. S___ seems to think there is no hope of my poor paralyzed man getting better, he may live for twenty years but can never walk. I am giving him English lessons every day. He is very quick at learning; it helps pass the time. Poor man, he has already been in bed six months.

March 21, 1915

This has been the most lovely spring day. The violets are blooming in the fields, they are smaller than ours but very fragrant; the yellow primroses are beautiful and grow everywhere. There is still lots of snow on the mountains but none in the valley. If it were not for the soldiers who are here we could scarcely believe that terrible fighting is going on so near us.

A lot of our men went off last week, some of them scarcely able to hobble, poor things, but all the hospitals are being cleared out to make room for the freshly wounded. We are expecting a new lot every day, and have prepared ten extra beds.

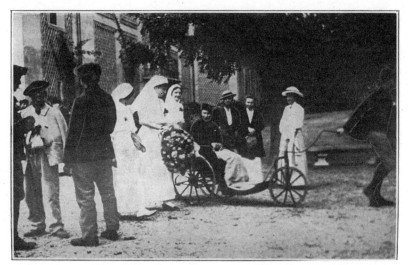

The hopelessly paralyzed man who afterwards walked
two miles on crutches. *My Beloved Poilus*

I will have some letters this week to send to the Red Cross and the De
Monts Chapter, I.O.D.E., thanking them for the things they sent back by
me; they have been so much appreciated, done so much good, and relieved
so much distress. I gave some to Mademoiselle de C___ who sent them
to a small hospital in Normandy near their chateau, some to the hospital
here, and some to a small hospital not far from here where they are very
poor; the doctor who is in charge there nearly wept when he knew the
things were for him.

March 26, 1915

Another beautiful day and the air is soft and balmy as a day in June.
The woods and fields are full of spring flowers, there are big soft gray
pussies on all the willow trees and the other trees are beginning to show
a faint tinge of green. It is certainly a lovely place.

You probably felt much relieved that I was not in Paris at the time of the last air raid when the bombs were dropped. One fell so near the ambulance at Neuilly that one of the doctors was knocked out of bed by the shock.

I had my paralyzed man out on the balcony today, it is the first time in six months that he has been out.

One of the men here, who has lost the use of both hands, told me today that he had six brothers in the army; two have been killed, two wounded, and two are still at the front. He was a coachman in a private family, has lost a thumb of one hand and on the other has only the thumb and one finger left. Fortunately his employer is a good man and will take care of him; but think of the poor man — horses are his chief joy, and he will never be able to drive again.

April 2, 1915

Easter Sunday and still raining. We had a splendid service from Mr. R____ and a Communion service after. The service is more like the Presbyterian than any other. We have four new soldiers but the large convoy has not yet arrived. There has been awful fighting in Alsace lately, so the wounded must come soon.

Today we had a specially good dinner for the men. Madam B___ gave them cigars and Easter eggs, and after dinner they sang some of their songs, then gave us three cheers. They are a fine lot of men and so grateful for everything we do for them.

The story of the dog has gone through the whole country, but it is nice to know that it is really true, and to have seen the dog.

Dr. B____ was able to save the other leg of the dog's master, and after another operation he thinks he will have the use of his hand.

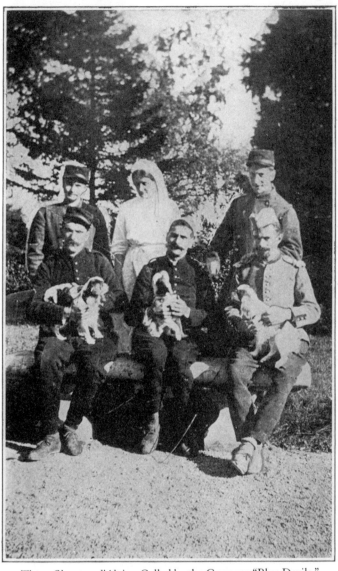

Three *Chasseurs d'Alpine*. Called by the Germans "Blue Devils."

My Beloved Poilus

April 10, 1915

We had a severe snow storm today and yesterday also, and in between the snow storms it poured rain; all the lovely spring weather has disappeared.

Wednesday night they announced the arrival of a train of wounded for the next morning at half-past five, but did not tell us how many to expect. We all went to the ambulance at half-past five and got everything ready for dressing and beds prepared for thirty. At seven thirteen arrived — all convalescents, and no dressings at all to do. The last time forty came, and all in a dreadful state of infection, so we never know what to expect.

I am not sorry I came back to Divonne for I feel that I have been able to help more here than in Paris; there they have many to help and here very few.

I am sending you a photo of three of my patients — *Chasseurs d'Alpine* or "Blue Devils" as the Germans call them — they are the ones who have done such wonderful work in Alsace.

April 19, 1915

I have had quite a busy week, for my men have been coming and going. The paralyzed man has been sent to Bourg, the two *Chasseurs d'Alpine* have gone and I have six new ones — this lot is ill, not wounded. There are three officers among them — one is a cousin of Madam B____, the French lady who helped establish this ambulance. Her husband came on Thursday; he has eight days leave. He is very interesting, for he has been all up through the north of France. He is adjutant to one of the generals and travels from eighty to one hundred miles a day in a motor, carrying despatches. There is a French aviator here, but he has not got his machine, so I am afraid there is no hope for me.

April 25, 1915

They took down all the stoves in the ambulance last week, and the day after it snowed; we had to put some of the men to bed to keep them warm. We have been very busy all week, new patients coming every day till now we have forty. Most of them are not wounded. Poor fellows, they are utterly done out; some have pneumonia, others rheumatism, one paralyzed and all sorts of other things. This is a wonderful place for them to come to and most of them get well very quickly. They are talking of increasing the number of beds in the hospital and of making it a regular military one. In that case they will send a military doctor here and the whole thing will be re-organized. They want me to promise to take charge of it, but I do not think it would be a wise thing, there is so much red tape and so many things about the military organization I do not understand, that I am afraid I would get into hot water at once.

I am sending you a circular of Mademoiselle de Caumont's lace school. They do lovely work and need all the help and orders that they can get. They will be glad to execute orders by mail for anyone writing them to Divonne-les-Bains, France.

May 2, 1915

I have never seen anything as lovely as the country is now, it is like one great garden; how I wish you could be here. I have had a busy day, as one of my patients had to be operated on. Dr. R___ took a piece of shrapnel out of his arm, and two others have been pretty ill; four leave tomorrow, so the general clearing up will begin again.

My poor old lady who had a stroke of paralysis died yesterday. I have been helping take care of her. The only son is at the front. So many old people are dying this year; when they get ill they don't seem to have any power of resistance; poor things, they have endured so much they cannot stand any more.

There is a poor little woman here who comes from Dinant that was destroyed by the Germans in the early part of the war.[2] She has lost all trace of her father and mother; her husband and brother have both been killed and their property utterly destroyed. Mr. B____, the pastor of the Protestant Church, has not been able to find his mother, who disappeared last August. Every day we hear of something new.

The papers are full of accounts of the gallant fighting of the Canadians, but the losses have been very heavy.[3]

May 9, 1915

It is just a year today since I sailed from New York, starting on our trip with Mrs. Eldridge. Little did we think of the horrors that have happened since.

Seven more men went off last night, so we have only twenty left. I have ten on my floor, but only four in bed; the others are able to be out all day. Charrel, one of my patients who just left, was one of six brothers, all of whom went off the first days of the war; three have been killed, the other three wounded.

I am going to Lyon on Thursday for a few days to visit some of the hospitals.

The French papers are full of the heroism of the Canadian troops; they have done wonderful work at Ypres, but at what a terrible cost.

I feel so proud every time I see the dressing gowns the De Monts Chapter sent me — they are the nicest we have.

---

[2] The town of Dinant in Belgium was destroyed by the Germans on August 23, 1914, and nearly seven hundred civilians killed.

[3] The 1st Canadian Division fought in the 2nd Battle of Ypres, April 22-26, during which it suffered more than six thousand casualties.

May 18, 1915

I left here Thursday at noon with Madam B____ who went to Paris. Before I left I telegraphed to Madam M____, the wife of the soldier who was here such a long time, asking her to get me a room, but when I arrived I found the whole family at the station to meet me and they insisted on my going home to stay with them. They are very simple people, but so kind and hospitable. I think it is quite an event having a stranger stay with them. We ate in the kitchen, and the whole family seemed to sleep in a cupboard opening off of it.

I saw a lot of hospitals and was rather favorably impressed with them. At the Hotel Dieu, they had received seven hundred patients within twenty-four hours. I think the saddest part was the eye ward, there were so many who would never see again and some of them so young. There were some with both legs gone and others both feet, and many with one arm or leg missing.

The boats on the river that were fitted up as hospitals were very interesting, but I fancy would be very hot in the summer and the mosquitoes would be terrible.

Saturday I spent the day with Mademoiselle R____, who had been staying at the hotel at Divonne for a time. The R____s are a wealthy family who have lived in Lyon for generations. Mademoiselle was able to take me to a good many of the hospitals, as they have done a good deal for them. We visited them in the morning, which was much more interesting, as we saw the work going on. At two of the hospitals wounded were arriving when we left there, so we saw the whole thing. I also saw the dressing being done in one of the large military hospitals. In the afternoon we went to a Red Cross hospital, where she worked in the *lingerie*; there are fifty beds and the patients are taken care of by the sisters. They seemed to be very cheerful and well looked after.

Sunday morning I got up at 3:30 and took a train at 4:30 for Romans where Mrs. C____ is working in a military hospital. At eight I arrived at Tournon and had to walk from there to a small village called Tain, where I got a tramway to Romans. I arrived at eleven, had my lunch on the sidewalk before a café — a most excellent meal for fifty cents. I found Mrs. C____ at the convent, where she is staying; fortunately she had the afternoon off. She has charge of the dressings and all of the infected operations. At the hospital where she is they have forty wounded Germans; they seem very contented and glad to be there. Mrs. C____ says it is dreadful to do their dressings, for they have no self-control at all; they have a certain dogged courage that makes them fight as they do in the face of certain death, but when they are wounded they cannot stand the pain. The French, on the contrary, seldom say a word; they will let one do anything, and if the pain is very bad they moan occasionally or say a swear word, but I have never seen one who lost control of himself and screamed.

I had dinner with Mrs. C____ at the convent, and at 7:15 took the train for Valence where I changed and waited two hours for the train to Lyon, but there was so much going on at the station that the time did not seem long — troops coming and going all the time and a hospital train with three hundred wounded arrived.

Monday morning I left for Divonne and arrived back very tired but well satisfied with my trip.

I found two new patients, one with a leg as big as an elephant and the other out of his head. I have twelve now on my floor.

Just think! Lily of the valley grows wild here, and you can get a bushel in a morning; the whole place is sweet with the perfume.

May 29, 1915

We got twelve more patients Wednesday — six left. I still have fifteen; this lot were all ill. One man is quite a character. The doctor put him on milk diet the first day — but he did not approve, so he went to the village and bought a loaf of bread and some ham.

Between the florist of the village and the wife of one of the soldiers I am kept well supplied with roses. I wish I could share my riches with you.

I am anxiously waiting to hear of the safe arrival of the 26th;[4] as we have heard nothing, they must be all right. It is hard to have them go but I cannot understand the attitude of those who will not go or who object to their men and boys going. You are just beginning to feel now what they have been suffering here since August last.

Madam L'H____ was called back to Verdun today; she was supposed to have three weeks' holidays, but has only been away ten days. She is not fit to go back but there is no help for it.

There was great excitement here when Italy finally declared war. It is awful to think of the brutes throwing bombs on Venice. I do hope they will not do any harm there.

I must say good-night, for I am tired. I am up at half-past five every morning and seldom get off duty before nine at night.

June 20, 1915

Yesterday we got five patients — the four worst were consigned to me. One poor chap was shot through the body and the spine was injured; they do not know just what the extent of the injury is, but he is completely paralyzed from the waist down. Fortunately he is very small, so it is not difficult to take care of him; he is the most cheerful soul, and says he has much to be thankful for as he has never suffered at all. When he was shot he simply had the sensation of his legs disappearing. When he fell he said to a comrade, "Both my legs have gone," but he had no pain at all. His comrade assured him that he had not lost his legs, but he said he could not believe it until he got to the hospital. He has received the *Médaille Militaire* for bravery, and his comrades said he certainly deserved it. He is so glad to get here, where it is real country and quiet. We put him on a *chaise longue* on the balcony today and he has been out of doors all day long.

It is after ten o'clock, but I am still at the ambulance. We are waiting for

---

4   The 26th (New Brunswick) Battalion, which was raised throughout the province, sailed from Saint John on June 13, 1915.

a train that is bringing us fifteen wounded directly from Alsace. Poor souls, they will be glad to get here, for they have been a long time on the way.

No letters this week; regulations are very strict again, and they are holding up all mail for eight or ten days.

June 22, 1915

I had to stop my letter as the men arrived. We got eighteen instead of fifteen. Such a tired dirty lot they were; they came straight from the battlefield, and had only had one dressing done since they were wounded. Some of them came on stretchers, others were able to walk, as they were wounded in the arms and head. I drew two from this lot, which brings my number up to seventeen again. One of mine has both bones broken in his leg and the other is wounded in the left side and shoulder. One poor chap had been a prisoner in one of the trenches for four days and they were unable to get any food all that time; most of them have slept ever since they arrived, they were so exhausted.

Today a military doctor came from Besançon to show us about some special electrical treatment. They are going to increase the beds by fifty to begin with, and later may make it three hundred.[5]

The news is not good to-day, the Russians seem to be retreating all the time and the losses in the north are terrible.

There seems to be no doubt in the minds of many people that the war will last another year at least; it seems too terrible.

June 27, 1915

I did not get my letter off today as there was so much to do. We have had inspection all week. They have finally decided to enlarge the hospital very much and make it a semi-military institution of four hundred beds.

---

[5] Throughout June 1915, the French army launched several secondary attacks along its front in support of its main offensive in May and June on Vimy Ridge, near Arras.

We are to turn the large dining-room into a ward with fifty beds, and the large part of the hotel will hold three hundred more. They want me to take charge. Dr. R___ will be chief with two assistants. There will be forty men nurses — convalescent soldiers — and I do not know how many more women nurses. I am very glad it has been so decided, for it is a great pity this place has not been of more use. Our last lot of men are getting on very well now; but we have had a hard week, for some of them were very ill. The doctor was very much afraid one man would lose his arm, but he has managed to save it.

I have grown to be a sort of official shotsnapper for the ambulance and village. It is really very interesting and my camera is very good.

Did I send you the snaps of the Bayin baby? She is only nine months old and runs around like a rabbit — is as pretty as a picture. I am so sleepy I can hardly see, so good-night.

July 4, 1915

I was glad to get your letter this week; three weeks on the way is a long time to wait.

I have such mixed feelings when I hear that the troops have left Saint John. My heart aches for those left behind, but I am so glad to know they are on the way, for they are needed badly and they will get a royal welcome, for Canadians have proved their worth. When they were in barracks and had nothing to do but drill they were not always angels; but when there was real work to be done their equal was not to be found. The French papers were full of the stories of their bravery. There were some officers who said that while others were splendid fighters the Canadians were marvelous.

It must have been terribly hard for Mrs.___ to let S___ go. I wish you would ask her for his address. I will try and get in touch with him and if he should be ill or wounded tell her I will go to him if I have to walk to get there. Get D___'s address also, so I can look after him. When I hear of them all being over here a wave of homesickness comes over me and I feel that I must go and join them.

There is much to be done on this side now, for the fighting in Alsace has been terrible. The last lot of soldiers that came were *Chasseurs d'Alpine*, and out of one thousand two hundred who went off only five hundred came back, and the greater number of them wounded.

Fifteen young men from this village have been missing since the terrible battle of three weeks ago, the deaths of a half a dozen have been confirmed but of the others nothing is known.

I am afraid there is no chance of the war finishing before the winter is over.

I wish somebody would organize a "French Day" or "Divonne Day" and collect pennies for me; we will need so many things before the winter is over. The general who came the other day said to make the money we have go to the furthest possible point, and then make debts — the soldiers must be taken care of.

July 11, 1915

We have had arrivals and departures all week. The days are not half long enough to do all that is necessary. My four men who came for electrical treatment are getting on wonderfully well, the big one who was paralyzed and who could not move hand or foot when he came, is now walking without crutches, and feeds himself.

The poor little *chasseur* who was shot through the body is really better. He is beginning to walk — with a great deal of help, of course. He can make the movements of walking and can put both legs straight out in front of him, and the doctor says there is great hope of a permanent cure. Poor little man, he deserves to get well, for I have never seen such courage and patience. We begin tomorrow to prepare the big dining room for fifty new patients, so we shall have a busy week. I am to have charge of the big ward and keep my floor as well. I will have two military men nurses and some more people from the village to help.

July 17, 1915

We have had a most terrific rain for the last two days — the people are getting anxious on account of the grain.

There was no celebration in the village on the fourteenth [Bastille Day] as is usual, but at the ambulance we had a little feast in honor of the men who were at Metzeral. We have four from the Seventh *Chasseurs*, whose regiment was decorated for unusual bravery.

My paralyzed man stood up alone last Sunday for the first time and now he walks, pushing a chair before him like a baby. He is the happiest thing you can imagine; for seven months he has had no hope of ever walking again.

Seven left last week and six more go on Monday, so we shall probably get a train load before long.

I have got a small English boy to help me in the mornings. He has been at school in Switzerland and the whole family have come here for the summer in order to help at the ambulance.

One of the great actors from Paris was here on Wednesday and played and sang for the men. He is making a tour in an automobile and visiting all the hospitals in order to give performances for the soldiers. A collection is taken up afterwards that goes towards the support of the hospital. The men were a most appreciative and enthusiastic audience.

There is a young Swiss doctor from Geneva here now who has come to help Dr. ___, who is very tired. I think he is rather surprised at the amount of work the old doctor gets through in a day. He said this morning that he would have to get up earlier in order to keep up with him.

The brother of my chambermaid has been missing for a month and the poor girl is terribly afraid he has been killed. He was at Arras, and the fighting there has been terrible.

Fifteen of the young men from the village are missing and every day comes the news of the death of someone.

We got five new men yesterday for electrical treatment; two of them are regular giants and we cannot get any clothes to fit them. They are devoted to my little paralyzed man, and sit around and watch him as if he was a baby just learning to walk.

I feel as sleepy as a dried apple tonight, so please forgive me if I tell you the same things over many times.

July 25, 1915

Miss Todd took me out in her motor today for an hour. We took Daillet, my star patient, with us. It was a pleasure to see his enjoyment. Dr. R___ was much surprised at the progress he had made in eight days; he says there is no doubt but that he will be entirely cured. Daillet wrote to his mother and told her that he could stand alone and was beginning to walk, but she did not believe it; she thought that he was just trying to cheer her up, so he asked me to take a photo of him standing up so that he could send it to her. He was the proudest, happiest thing you can imagine when he sent it off. Then his aunt came to see him, so the poor mother is finally convinced that it is true, and is coming to see him as soon as the haying is done, but she has to work in the fields now and cannot get away.

It is wonderful the work that the women do here. There are only two old horses left in the whole village, so the women harness themselves into the rakes and wagons, and pull them in place of the horses — and they so seldom complain of the hard work. I asked one woman if she did not find it very hard, and she said at first it came very difficult but she got used to it and it was nice to be able to do their part.

We got twenty men from Alsace on Friday — some of them badly wounded. They did not arrive till half-past eleven at night, and it was three in the morning before we got the dressings done and got them to bed. It is the second time that some of them have been wounded. They are all *Chasseurs d'Alpine* — they are a splendid type. Some of them had both legs and both arms wounded. Yesterday we were rather anxious about several of them, but today they are better. They generally sleep about three days after they arrive, they are so done out.

Mrs. H____ has had to leave to care for a typhoid patient, so my hands are very full. My English boy is getting trained rapidly; he is only seventeen and not very strong, too young to go to the war but very keen to do something to help.

Do not worry about me, I am as well as possible and as strong as a horse, but as my day begins at half-past five in the morning and ends at half-past nine at night I fall asleep over my letters.

Thanks for the clippings; I would not have known Bayard [Warner's nephew] if the name had not been there. I do not dare to think of his coming, and yet I would not be proud of him if he did not want to come. I shall try and get up to the north later so as to be nearer him when he comes.

Good-night, mother; these are sad times, but we must not lose courage. I wish I could see you to-night.

August 1, 1915

To say that I was delighted will not express my feelings when I got the letter from the Loyalist Chapter, I.O.D.E., enclosing cheque. It was awful good of them to help us here, for I realize the demands for help on every side and it is only natural that they should send to the Canadians first. But Oh! it is so badly needed and will so do much good here. I had been racking my brain trying to think of a way to scratch up a few pennies, and then this delightful surprise came.

This hospital is called the "Paradise of the Seventh Region," for it is so very far ahead of most of the French military hospitals. But while there is a good deal of luxury on one side, such as pleasant airy rooms, comfortable beds, good food and air, on the other hand there is a great lack of what we consider necessities. The first thing I did when I got the letter with the money was to order a foot tub for each floor, slippers for the patients when they are in the house, scissors for the pharmacy and for each floor, and various other small things that I have been longing for and that will save many steps. Now that the capacity of the hospital has been increased by fifty beds, it is more difficult than ever to get money from the general fund for things of that kind; it really has to be kept for food and heating. We also need instruments and basins, etc., for a table for dressings in the new ward, as we have absolutely nothing. Then it is so nice to have a fund that we can draw on in case of need. Sometimes the men are terribly poor and cannot afford to get anything for themselves when they leave. Sometimes a ticket for a wife or daughter to come to see them and cheer them up. It is the second time some of these men have been wounded and they have not seen their families for a year.

It is just a year today (August 1) since mobilization began. At five o'clock in the morning the tocsin sounded and all the village gathered at the town hall to read the notice of mobilization. There were many sad and anxious hearts then, but many more now, for there is not a family who has not lost someone who is near and dear·to them — and still it goes on. I wonder when the end will come.

My prize patient, Daillet, walks down stairs by himself now by holding on to the railing like a child. We are all proud of him. The doctor who sent him here from Besançon came in the other day to see how he was getting on and he could not believe it when he saw him.

I am almost asleep so I must stop. I made a mistake this morning, got up at half-past four instead of half-past five.

August 15, 1915

In the face of all the terrible things which are happening one must not worry over little things. I have got to the stage now when I feel as if one should never complain or worry if they have a roof over their heads and enough to eat, and that all one's efforts should be given to helping others.

I feel perfectly overwhelmed with the letters that ought to be written, but cannot find time to do them. I have been up all night and a couple of days. We got thirty new patients last night. They arrived at 3 a.m. and it was half-past five before we got them to bed. I did not get any of this lot, as my rooms were full. There were not so many wounded — more sick, rheumatism, bronchitis, etc. One poor man said it was like going directly from hell to heaven; it was the first time he had slept in a bed for a year

It is nearly eleven and I must be up early, so good-night.

August 23, 1915

Your letter has been long delayed, as they are very strict and holding up the mails again.

We heard this morning that there are French troops guarding the border at Crassier, just half a mile from here. We hear all the Swiss border is to be protected by barbed wire. I do not know what it all means unless it is on account of spies.

We got fifteen more patients last week, one yesterday and one today, but as several went away we have still the same number — eighty-four.

We have had a very busy morning. An inspector arrived just as we were ready to operate, and between the two I did not know whether I was on my head or my heels. Thirty of our men will go off on Monday and we will probably get a train full later in the week.

We have a phonograph with a rasping voice that plays from morning to night. The soldiers love it; the poor things are so used to noise that they don't seem happy without it, but sometimes I feel as if I could scream.

One of the men got a telegram saying his mother was dying; the doctor gave him forty-eight hours leave — all he could possibly do — so he went home and has just got back; could not stay for the funeral, but was so thankful to have been able to see her. If he had been at the front that would not have been possible — only another sad consequence of the war. Another soldier received the news of the death of his little girl.

Miss Todd took me out in her motor the other day. We had a beautiful run over the mountains; the view was magnificent. We took one of the soldiers with us and he enjoyed himself immensely; it was the first time he had ever been in one.

August 29, 1915

It is pouring rain, it is sad to say, as the soldiers are having a little celebration. A band came from Nejon and the Count de Divonne made a speech, two of the men received their *Croix de Guerre*, the doctor made such a nice little speech to each of them. It was very touching to see the groups of men, some with arms in slings and others with legs and heads bandaged, and some who could not stand at all, still others were in their beds. The decorations were given in the *Grand*[e] *Salle*.

I am not sure if all your letters reach me or not, sometimes I get two in a week and then again none for three weeks.

Thirty-three men go off tomorrow, some of them cured and back to the front, some who will never be better, and some to go home on convalescence.

Today the florist in the village sent a clothes basket full of roses to the Ambulance for the fete. I thought of you and wished you could have some.

September 5, 1915

Thanks for the money you sent from a friend in your last letter. I will use it wisely and make it go as far as possible. There will be more suffering this winter than there was last, but they are so brave, these people, they seldom complain of anything.

There is a little woman here whose husband was killed. She makes twenty cents a day selling papers and gets ten cents a day pension. She has three children, the eldest a girl of twelve. I got her a good pair of boots the other day and warm underclothes for the other children. She was so grateful.

Don't worry about me. My expenses are very small, I have not bought any clothes and do not need any this winter.

Today they had a big concert in the hotel, the proceeds go to the ambulance.

We have had an awful week of rain and cold, but hope for a little more sunshine to thaw us out.

Our good doctor is going to be married next month. I am so glad, for he lives all alone and needs some one to look after him.

I shall have to go to bed to get warm. There is no heat in this house and when it rains it is like an ice box.

September 11, 1915

I expect to leave here in two weeks to go to an ambulance at the front. It is somewhere in the north in Belgium. I think Dr. R___ is sorry to have me leave, but it will be a much larger field and the kind of a place where there will be much to do. They have all been so nice to me here about helping me get my papers ready to send to the minister of war, so I do not think there will be any difficulty in my getting through. I go to Paris first, then to Dunkirk, where Mrs. T___ [Mary Borden Turner?] will meet me, after that my destination is uncertain. Do not worry if you do not hear from me regularly, for it may be difficult to get mail through. I will write as usual.

I cannot tell you how glad I am to be able to go to the front, for it means a chance to do good work and I shall be so glad to be in the north when Bayard comes over and nearer the Canadian boys. Even if I cannot see them I shall not feel so far away.

One of my men today got word that his baby, seven months old, had just died and the little girl of two is very ill. He expected to go next week and has been counting the days till he could see them. He has never seen the baby as it was born after the war began — another one of the sad things of this awful war.

Good-night; I am so glad of the chance of active service.

September 19, 1915

My orders came today, and I leave on Tuesday for Paris and on Friday for Dunkirk. I am up to my eyes in work, for there is so much to be done before leaving and new people to break in. Three military nurses arrived yesterday, but it is rather difficult to manage for they know nothing at all about taking care of sick people. They have all been at the front, and wounded too badly to return and sent into an auxiliary service. One is a priest, one a hair dresser, and the third a horse dealer; however, they are nice men and are willing to learn, which is a great thing in their favour.

If they are able to raise any money for me I will see that it is wisely spent. There is great need everywhere, and I am proud of the people of Saint John, they have done so much.

There is a poor woman who lives in a little village near here. She had two sons — one has been killed in the war, the other a helpless cripple for eighteen years and is not able to move out of his chair. He makes baskets sometimes, but now there is no one to buy the baskets. The mother goes out by the day but can earn so little. I gave him five francs, one of the De Monts dressing gowns, and some warm underclothes. He was so grateful, poor boy, and says he will not feel the cold now. His mother is away nearly all day and he sits by the window all alone and depends upon the neighbours coming in to help him from time to time; he is always cheerful and never complains.

The W___s have such a hard time — they get so little of their income since the war began. It has gradually gone down from $3,000 per year to $500; four of them to live on that amount. So many people are in just the same condition, there is no end to the misery.

I do not know whether it is the French or the English army we are to follow at my new post.

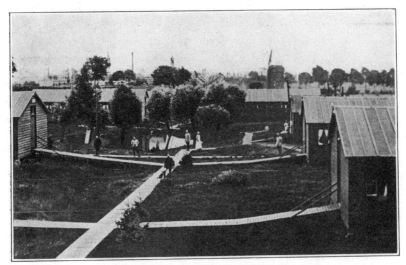

Ambulance Volant, France. *My Beloved Poilus*

September 23, 1915
Paris

I am off tomorrow at 7:30 a.m., to Boulogne, then Calais, and reach Dunkirk at 9:30 p.m.

I have had two very strenuous days and will be glad to rest in the train tomorrow. It took such a time to get my papers in order. The thermometer for the last two days has been about 100.

Mobile No. 1,
France

I am really not in France but Belgium. I cannot tell you just where, but it is within ten miles of the firing line, and not far from the place where so many of our boys from home have been sent. I thought when I came here that it would be entirely English, as the lady who gave the hospital is an American married to an Englishman. The English are not far away but they are taken to their own hospitals.

We belong to a little wedge of the French that is in between the English and Belgians. It is a regular field hospital and is composed of a great many portable huts or sheds; some are fitted up as wards, another the operating room, another the pharmacy, another supply room, laundry, nurses' quarters, doctors' quarters, etc. It is a little colony set down in the fields and the streets are wooden sidewalks.

The first night I arrived I did not sleep, for the guns roared all night long, and we could see the flashes from the shells quite plainly; the whole sky was aglow. The French and English guns sounded like a continuous roar of thunder; but when the shells from the German guns landed on this side we could feel a distinct shock, and everything in our little shanty rattled.

Yesterday I saw my first battle in the air between German and French aeroplanes. We could scarcely see the machines, they were so high up in the air, but we could see the flashes from their guns quite distinctly and hear the explosion of the shells. Today a whole fleet of aeroplanes passed over our heads; it was a wonderful sight.

There are about one hundred and fifty beds in all here.

I have been inspected by doctors, captains, generals, and all kinds of people till I am weary. I hope they are satisfied at last, but I cannot go off the hospital grounds until I have two different kinds of passes given to me — one is a permission to go on the roads about here and the other is good as far as Dunkirk.

We have a man in our ward who had a piece of shrapnel the size of an egg in his abdomen; they had to take out about half a yard of intestines, which had been torn to pieces. He was also shot through the shoulder, in the arm and leg. As we got him within two hours after he was wounded there was no infection, and having a clever surgeon he is getting along famously. Another poor chap has lost his right arm and shot through the liver as well as being cut up by a piece of shrapnel — he is getting well also. Two have died, and it is a blessing; for to live in darkness the rest of one's life is worse than death. The Germans are using a new kind of gas bomb that blinds the men.

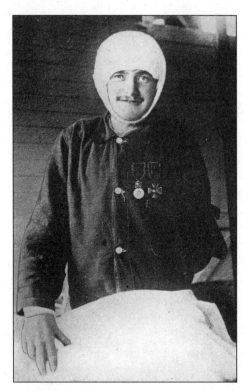

Thought to be a hopeless case.
But everyone must have their
chance, three doctors operated
at once, amputating leg,
an arm and trepanning.
Now as happy as the day is long.
My Beloved Poilus

It is pouring rain tonight and cheerless enough here, but I can only think of the poor men in the trenches.

I got a joyful surprise today — a letter from Mr. Bell enclosing a post office order from Mr. Calhoun of Philadelphia. Nothing gives me so much pleasure as to help these poor people.

It is beginning to get cold. I shall get bed socks for the men, for they have not enough hot water bags to go round and all suffer from cold feet.

I passed Colonel MacLaren's hospital in the train — it is very impressive to see the rows and rows of white tents. I also saw some Canadian nurses in the distance, and did so want to get out and speak to them.

I must go to bed now to get warm. As long as one keeps going the cold is not so apparent but when one sits still it is not pleasant.

There are four English, three American, and three French nurses here.

October 3, 1915

My fund is like the widow's cruse — it never gives out. Somebody is always sending me something. I do hope they all realize how grateful I am and how much good I have been able to do. I have been very careful how I spent it.

A boy of twenty went off today. He had absolutely nothing warm to put on him, so I got him an outfit at Dunkirk. He was almost blown to pieces, poor boy, and he said that one sock was all that was left of his clothes. They provide them with necessary things at the hospital, but sometimes the supply gets a bit low and now it is so cold they need extra underclothing. When he was brought in they put him in a ward by himself because they thought he would not live through the night, he was so terribly wounded. His right arm was gone, he had a bullet in his liver — it is still there — and multiple wounds of head and body. But he made a wonderful recovery and went away very white and weak, but cheerful and confident that he will get something to do that will not require two hands. He has the *Médaille Militaire* and the *Croix de Guerre*, and his lieutenant, captain, and general have all been to see him several times — they say he was a wonderful soldier.

Three of us went to Dunkirk by motor to get various supplies. We saw many interesting things on the way, and in Dunkirk saw the destruction caused by the bombardment. The whole side was out of the church and several houses were simply crushed like a pack of cards. Some of the nurses were in Dunkirk when it was bombarded, and they said the noise was the most terrifying part of it all.

The day we went to Dunkirk we saw a lot of armoured cars. Such curious looking things they are — some are painted with blotches of yellow and green and gray and red and brown so they cannot be distinguished from the landscape. We saw lots of English troops. I looked in vain for Canadians, but they are not far off.

It has been awfully cold so far and rains most of the time. We have decided that we shall just keep putting on clothes like the Italians do in winter and never take anything off.

We get wounded every day, sometimes not more than half a dozen, but as they are almost all seriously wounded we are kept busy.

There have been so many troops moving on lately that we thought we would be left without anything to do. We have orders not to do anything that is not absolutely necessary as we may have to move also.

I believe the hospital at Divonne has been taken over by the nuns. I miss the lovely flowers that I had there. I share a small room with two other nurses and there is not much room to spare. We have boxes put up on end for tables and wash stands, and there is only one chair. Some of the nurses have tents, two in each.

We have had a terrible busy week. All the new ones that came into my ward lived only thirty-six or forty-eight hours — they were too far gone to save. Five went away cured and they really were cases to be proud of.

I think it was the sweetest thing of little Mary Murray to send me her birthday money for my soldiers. I have been getting them fruit and cigarettes for Sunday. That is the thing that overwhelms me at times — the awful suffering every way one turns. Dorothy Thompson sent me £5, much to my joy.

Last night I could not sleep for the noise of the guns; they must have been bombarding some place near at hand, for the whole earth seemed to shake.

The boys who drive the American ambulance and bring our patients in say this place is a sort of heaven to them, they are always glad to get here. Mrs. T___ [Turner?] does everything she can for them. They are a nice lot of boys and are doing good work.

Some of the poor men who have lost large pieces of their intestines find the hospital diet a little hard.

November 7, 1915
Mobile No. 1

Letter writing is done under difficulties here. I have gone to bed in order to keep warm and have a small lantern with a candle in to light the paper.

November 15, 1915

I did not get any further with my letter for the kitty insisted upon playing with the candle and I was afraid we would have a fire, and since then I have been so busy I have not had a minute. We have had three glorious days and have appreciated them, I can tell you. It has been so cold and wet we have all been water-logged. As for me, I have no word to express my gratitude for all the friends have sent to me. I am quite overwhelmed with all the gifts of money and supplies, but I shall make good use of them and nothing shall be wasted.

The wool which Mrs. S___ sent turned up yesterday and I have already given half of it to the women in one of the villages here to knit into socks. There is a dear old English colonel who has a soup kitchen near the firing line and he is always looking for socks. He does a great deal of good, for he gets the men when they are carried in from the trenches and gives them hot drinks and hot water bottles, and warm socks when he has them. So many of the men have just straw in their boots and are almost frozen. It makes such a difference if they can get warmed up quickly. Poor souls, they have had a hard time since the heavy rains began. They are brought in here just caked with mud from head to foot.

Oh, how glad I was to get the cheque from the Red Cross Society and the cheque from Miss G___. I have written to her and would like to write long letters to everyone who is so kind, but there is not time.

This ambulance was established by an American lady who then gave it to the French government. The expenses of running it are paid by them, but I think Mrs. Mary Borden Turner pays the nurses and also helps out in the way of extra supplies.

On All Saints Day we went to the little cemetery and decorated the graves of the soldiers who have died in the hospital. There was a special mass and service in the churchyard and the general sent us an invitation. It was pouring rain but I would not have missed it for anything, and I only wish the mothers, wives, and sisters could know how beautiful it all was and how tenderly cared for are the last resting places of their dear ones. It was a picture I shall never forget. The corner of the little churchyard with the forty new graves so close together, each marked with a small wooden cross and heaped high with flowers — the general standing with a group of officers and soldiers all with bared heads — the nurses and one or two of the doctors from the hospital behind them, and then the village people and refugees — hundreds of them, it seemed to me — and the priest giving his lesson — and all the time the rain coming down in torrents and nobody paying any attention to it. There were no dry eyes, and when the general came and shook hands with us afterwards, he could not speak. He is a splendid man, very handsome and a patriot to the backbone — one of the finest types of Frenchmen.

Do not worry about me for I am very well and so glad to be here in spite of the cold and discomforts. Mrs. S____'s socks and bandages have just come.

November 28, 1915

It is bitterly cold here and we feel it more because it is so damp. I can't tell you how thankful I am to be able to get socks and warm things for the men. We can send things to the first dressing station by the ambulances and from there they go to the trenches at once. Mrs. D____'s socks came yesterday, and I sent them off to Colonel Noble, who has the soup kitchen at the front. All Mrs. S____'s have been given away. It was such a good idea to have them white, for they put them on under the others and it often saves the men from being infected by the dye of the stockings.

This morning when I got up my room was like a skating pond, for the moisture had frozen on the floor and the water in the pitcher was solid.

The getting up in the morning is the hardest, but after we get started we do not mind the cold.

The patients have plenty of blankets and hot water bottles, so they do not suffer.

Two Zeppelins went over our head yesterday, but fortunately we are too unimportant to be noticed. I suppose that is one of the reasons they will not let us say where we are, for there are so many spies everywhere that can send information.

An English nurse came yesterday; she has had most interesting experiences. She was in Brussels when it was taken by the Germans and was obliged to take care of German soldiers and officers for some time. She said the officers, as a rule, were brutes, but some of the men were very nice and grateful.

For three days and nights the guns have thundered without ceasing. I wonder what it all means?

My kitty keeps all the seventeen dogs that loaf around here in order. Yesterday she chased a big yellow dog, half St. Bernard, down the main sidewalk of the ambulance. It was a very funny sight, for she was like a little round ball of fury and the poor dog was frightened to death.

December 5, 1915

Last night we had the most awful wind storm. I thought our little hut would be carried over into the German lines. It rained in torrents and the roof leaked, and I could not get my bed away from the drips, so I put up my umbrella and the kitty and I had quite a comfortable night.

Ben Ali, the poor Arab who was so desperately wounded, was up today for the first time.

I have ordered six dozen pair of socks from Paris. My nice old English Colonel Noble (with the soup kitchen) is always clamouring for them. I think he saves lots of the men from having frozen feet.

December 26, 1915

Christmas is over, and in spite of the undercurrent of sadness and the suffering the men had a very happy day. In my ward all but one were well enough to enjoy the tree, and they were like a lot of children with their stockings. Christmas Eve one of the orderlies who was on guard helped me decorate the ward and trim the tree, then we hung up their stockings. They had oranges, sweets, and cigarettes, and some small toys and puzzles and various things of that kind to amuse them.

I had a package for each one in the morning, and, thanks to my good friends at home, was able to give them some nice things. I had a pair of warm socks and gloves for each one, a writing pad and envelopes, pen, pencil, small comb in a case, tooth brush, tooth powder, piece of soap, wash cloth, and a small alcohol lamp with solidified alcohol — a thing made especially for the trenches and which delighted them very much — also a small box of sweets, and to several of the very poor ones I gave a small purse with five francs in it. One poor boy said he had never had such a Christmas in his life; he is one of a family of seven, and says that in times of peace it was all they could do to get enough to eat.

Christmas day at four o'clock the tree was lighted, and one of the many priests who acts as an *infirmier* (male nurse) here came round to the different wards and sang carols. He has a very beautiful voice and was much appreciated by the soldiers. Mrs. Turner then came in, followed by an orderly with a huge hamper containing a present for each man. They had a wonderful dinner, soup, raw oysters (which came from Dunkirk by motor), plum pudding, etc. I could only give my men a bite of pudding to taste it, but they were able to eat the oysters and other things in moderation.

In the other wards, where there were only arms and legs and heads to consider, they had a royal feast. She also gave a grand dinner to all the *infirmiers* and men on the place — had a tree for them and a present for each one. We also had a good dinner and a present for each. She certainly went to a great deal of trouble and made many people happy.

The next day we divided the things on the trees and each man made a package to send home to his children. They were even more delighted to be able to do this than with their own things.

One poor man in my ward was so ill that I was afraid he would die, so I moved his bed to the end of the ward and put screens around it so that he would not be disturbed, and that the others would not be disheartened by seeing him. He was so much better Christmas night that we had great hopes of saving him, but today he died. He was wounded in seven places and one hip was gone. The general came at four o'clock and decorated him. He roused up and saluted and seemed so pleased. In the evening the doctor came to do his dressing and he seemed much better. After the doctor had gone he turned to me and said, "that major knows what he is about, he is a corker."

Ben Ali, my prize Arab, had a wonderful day. He ate too much and had to stay in bed today, but he has been wrapping and unwrapping his presents and having a fine time. He is just like a child, he is so pleased. He has taken a great fancy to me and asked me to visit him after the war is over.

We had midnight mass on Christmas eve for the *infirmiers* and personnel of the hospital. One of the empty wards was fitted up as a chapel and a Franciscan monk from Montreal officiated. He is on duty here in the *lingerie* and is a splendid man. He is delicate, has some serious heart trouble, so that he need not stay, but he came over to do what he could for his country and his services are invaluable here. His mother was in the north of the country taken by the Germans and he has not been able to get any news of her for more than a year.

We have had orders from headquarters to close all the shutters as soon as the lights are lit, so we feel as if we were shut up in packing cases.

There were a great many aeroplanes flying about today, so I suppose they are expecting an attack of some kind. It is blowing a gale tonight and I feel as if our little shanty would blow over.

January 1, 1916

It is hard to believe that we are beginning another year. If only it will bring a lasting peace! The boxes have not turned up yet, but they doubtless will one of these days, and we will be all the more glad to see them because we have used up everything else.

I expected to go on night duty immediately after Christmas, but we had such sick people in my ward they did not want to make a change just then.

It is blowing a gale again tonight, and raining in torrents; it seems as if it would never stop raining. The roof of one of the wards was loosened the other night the wind was so strong, so the patients had to be all moved out while it was being mended. Our barracks had to be propped up also, all one side was loose and the rain came in sheets. I frequently go to bed with an umbrella.

January 16, 1916

We have had orders to evacuate all the men who are able to travel, so we got rid of a great many — eighteen went on Tuesday, twenty on Friday, and nineteen more are to go next Tuesday.

The roof nearly blew off my ward last night, so my patients had to be moved into the next ward till it is mended. I am going to take advantage of it and have a thorough house cleaning.

Le Roux, the boy who has been here so long and who has been so terribly ill, died on Tuesday. I had great hopes of him up till the last day. Half an hour after he died the general came to decorate him. I hope they will send the medals to his people; it seems hard that they should have been just too late to give them to him. The next day I went to his funeral — the first soldier's funeral I have seen. I was impressed with the dignity and simplicity of it. The plain deal coffin was covered with a black pall, which had a white cross at the head, the French flag covered the foot and a bunch of purple violets, tied with red, white, and blue ribbon, lay between.

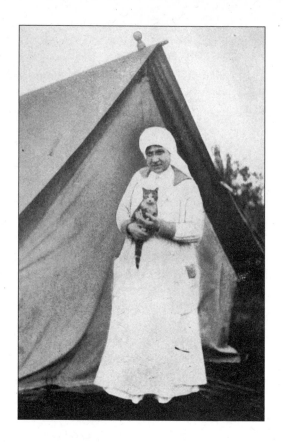

Nurses' quarters for two.
My Beloved Poilus

It was carried in one of the covered military carts. At three o'clock the little procession started for the cemetery. First came the priest in soldier's uniform, carrying a small wooden cross, on which was written Le Roux's name and the name of his regiment. One of this kind is always put at the head of each grave. Then came three soldiers with guns on their shoulders, then the car bearing the coffin, and on each side three soldiers with arms reversed; directly behind were two *infirmiers* and three soldiers with guns on their shoulders, we two nurses in our uniforms, then two officers and some more soldiers. As we went down the road to the little church in R____ [Rousbrugge?] we passed long lines of soldiers going somewhere, and everyone saluted. A few stray people followed us into the church and afterwards to the graveyard, where we left Le Roux with his comrades who had gone before. I had not been there since All Saints Day and it was sad to see how many more graves had been added to the line. The ward seems very empty without Le Roux, but I am glad that the poor boy is at rest for he has suffered so long. I am beginning to think that death is the only good thing that can come to many of us.

January 25, 1916

We have been awfully busy, wounded arriving every night, sometimes nine and sometimes ten, etc. Tonight we have had only six so far, but will probably have some more before eight a.m., they have all been very bad cases. There has been a terrific bombardment every night we have been on duty.

My little tent nearly blew away in the big wind storm, so I had to sleep in the barracks — or rather try to sleep. I did not succeed very well, so today I moved back to the tent. From my bed in the tent I can see the troops passing on the road and aeroplanes in the sky. Today we saw so many we knew it would mean trouble tonight. The trenches were bombarded, and some of the poor men who were wounded had to lie in the mud and cold for over twelve hours before they could be moved, consequently they arrived here in a pretty bad shape. One of the men had on a pair of Mrs. D___'s socks. I had sent them to Colonel Noble and he gave them to the men in the trenches. It has been clear and frosty for two nights, such a relief after all the rain. The hospital is full of very sick men. I am glad to be on night duty for a change.

January 30, 1916

It has been so cold and damp today that I could not get warm, even in bed. I like sleeping out in the little tent and as a rule sleep very well — have a cup of hot tea when they wake us at six o'clock. I wear two pair of socks, besides the rooms are not so frightfully damp since we got up the little stoves; they get dried out once a day, which is a great advantage.

I am sending you some snap shots of my little kitty. We call her "Antoinette" after the aeroplane, for she makes a noise like the aeroplane when she sings.

When I have a chance I shall go back to Divonne for a rest — it is too far to go home — but there does not seem any chance of it at present. The English nurses who have been here six months will have to go first, and we are more than busy. There are two new nurses coming next week — Canadians, I think. It is very difficult to get nurses up here, there is so much red tape to go through.

You must not worry about me, for I am really very well. The cold and simple life is very healthy, even if it is not always comfortable. I seem to be as strong as an ox and the more I have to do the better I feel.

It is joyful to hear that I am to have some more money. Saint John people certainly have been good. A box came today from Trinity, it had been opened. There is the ambulance, I must run.

February 6, 1916

We are so busy here that we scarcely know where to turn. It is just a procession of wounded coming and going all the time, for we have to send them off as quickly as possible in order to make room for the new arrivals. Thirty-eight went off last Tuesday and fifteen on Friday, but the beds are filled up again. The last ones we have been getting are so badly wounded that I wonder who can be moved on Tuesday. We have had wild wind and rain for the last week, but today is cold and clear, and for the first time in weeks it is quiet — the cannonading has been incessant.

Two English aviators were brought in yesterday whose machine fell quite near here; fortunately they are not very badly hurt.

The box from the high school girls came today, and it was like having Christmas all over again — such a nice lot of things there were. I shall have a fine time distributing them.

Here comes the ambulance. One poor man died in the receiving ward and the other two went to the operating room at once. They both have symptoms of gas gangrene, and I am afraid one will lose an arm and the other a leg.

In spite of the cold and wet we keep extraordinarily well.

Four new nurses have come, much to our relief, for the work was getting rather beyond us. Two of them are Canadians from Toronto. They know ever so many people I know. They sailed from Saint John at Christmas time and saw so many Saint John friends of mine — they said everyone was so good to them.

We do not get a minute during the night and some days have been up to lunch time.

February 22, 1916

There have been two big attacks and we have had our hands full. Since Sunday the cannonading has gone on without ceasing. It seems to be all round us. At night we can see the flashes of the guns quite distinctly, in fact the sky is lit up most of the time. It is like the reflection of a great fire — it would be very beautiful if one could get away from the horror of what it all means.

The aeroplanes were almost as thick as the motors — one came down in a field near the hospital yesterday — the wings were riddled with bullets, but fortunately the aviator was not hurt. We often see Taubes [German aircraft], and Zeppelins have gone over us several times, though I could not recognize them, but the noise was unmistakable. The wounded are nearly all brought in at night so we have our hearts and hands full. The other night twenty-three came in at once so we had to call up the day people to help us; seventeen were operated upon and all are getting well but one.

From July 23, 1915, until January 1, 1916, seven hundred and fifty patients have been cared for here and sixty-six have died. I have had over one hundred wounded come in at night this last month, and as they all come directly from the trenches you can imagine what it means.

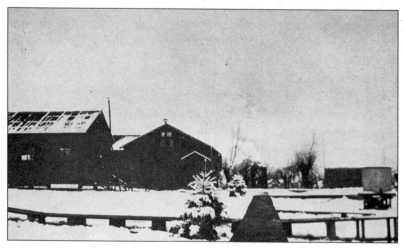

Ambulance Volant in winter. *My Beloved Poilus*

Such a fine box came from Mrs. S___ and F___ containing bandages, socks, etc., all most welcome.

The ground is white with snow today but it will not stay long.

It is very difficult to get nurses here as a command of the French language is an essential.

The guns are still at it, so there will be much to do tonight.

March 6, 1916

We have had snow several times this week and it is snowing again today. It is very pretty for a little while but soon melts, and the mud is worse than ever.

I feel that I can never be grateful enough to the people who have enabled me to do so much for these poor men. I am going to order some more pillows, they are things that we need very much. All the lung cases have to sit up in bed and need a great many pillows to make them comfortable. Strange to say we have not lost a lung case and we have had some pretty bad ones. There is one in now who was shot through the lung, and yesterday they took out a long sibber bullet [?] from under his rib; he will be able to go home next week. When he came in he was in very bad condition and he could not speak for a week. The treatment is to sit them up in bed and give them morphine every day to keep them perfectly quiet, the hemorrhage gradually stops, and they get well very quickly. We have had a number of deaths from that awful gas gangrene; there is not much hope when that attacks them.

The bombardments have been so terrible lately that those who are wounded in the morning cannot be taken out of the trenches until night, and then they are in a sad condition.

One day last week, just as I was getting ready to go to bed, some people came out from the village to ask if we could help a poor girl who had been burned. Mrs. Turner and I went at once with all sorts of dressings and found her in a terrible state — her whole body burned — so of course there was no hope. She only lived three days. I went in the mornings to do her dressing and another nurse in the afternoon. She was burned by lighting a fire with oil.

Things are too heavy now for me to get my holiday.

March 12, 1916

Only ten admissions. All the efforts are being directed against Verdun.[6] The defence has been magnificent, and if only the ammunition holds out there will be no danger of the Germans getting through; but what a terrible waste of good material on both sides.

Mrs. Turner has been obliged to go to Paris and has left me in charge of the hospital. I hope nothing terrible will happen while she is away.

The snow is all gone and we are having rain again.

My kitty is getting very bad and spends all her nights out. She has grown to be just a common ordinary cat now, but she caught a rat the other day, so has become useful instead of ornamental.

---

6   The Germans launched a major offensive against the French at Verdun on February 21, 1916. The campaign lasted until December.

March 20, 1916

I am left in charge of the ambulance for a time and am a bit nervous, having French, English, American, Canadian, and Australian nurses under me.

We had quite an exciting time yesterday watching a German being chased by four French machines. They all disappeared in the clouds so we do not know what happened. Today I counted eleven aeroplanes in the air at once as well as three observation balloons. One aeroplane came so close over the barracks that we could wave to the pilot.

We had a lot of patients out of doors today, some on stretchers, others on chairs, and others had their beds carried out — they enjoyed it so much. We take advantage of all the good weather.

It is pouring again tonight and the guns are booming in an ominous manner.

One day last week I went to Poperinghe with Mrs. C___. We heard there [were] some Canadian troops there and I was hoping to find some friends, but the Canadians had been moved; however, we talked with some Tommies, gave them cigarettes and chocolate, and had a very interesting time.

March 29, 1916

Just a week ago a French general was brought in wounded in the leg while he was inspecting the Belgian trenches. We were rather overwhelmed at first, but I arranged a corner of one of the wards and he spent one day and night there while we fixed up an empty ward for him. The next day his wife arrived and she is camping quite contentedly in another corner of the ward. She, poor woman, has suffered much from the war but is very brave. Her eldest son was killed, her second son is ill at Amiens, and this is the second time the general has been wounded. The first time he was in a hospital for three months. Her nephew, who is like a second son, has also been killed, and his wife, a young woman of twenty-two, taken prisoner by the Germans, and they have had no news of her since

September, 1914. The general's home was in the Aisne district and is, of course, in the hands of the Germans. There is nothing left of the house but the four walls; everything has been packed off to Germany, all the wood work and metal has been taken for the trenches. The day the general was brought in, the King of the Belgians came to decorate him, and we were all so disappointed because we did not know about it and only one or two of us saw him. He came in a motor, accompanied only by one officer, and we did not know anything about it until he had gone.

We had another awful storm last night — wind and rain. Windows blew off and doors blew in, and one poor little night nurse was blown off the sidewalk and nearly lost in the mud.

One day last week I was surprised by a visit from two Canadian boys. They were doing some engineering work in this section and when they heard there were Canadians here they came over to see us. One was from Toronto, the other from Fort William. I gave them one of the Christmas cakes and some cigarettes. They went away very happy. I was hoping to get news of some of our boys, but they did not know any of them personally but expected to see some of the men from the 26th Battalion in a few days. I told them to tell any who could to come and see us. I have been hoping ever since their visit to see Bayard or S___ or D___ walk in some day. It is awful to know that they are so near and not be able to see them.

April 8, 1916

.   A cheque came today from the De Monts Chapter, I.O.D.E., which gave me great joy. It touches me to tears to think of the way the Saint John people have helped me. I wish they could have a look in here and see how much more I have been able to do on account of the help they have sent me.

There is a soldier who helps here by the name of Baquet; his wife has just taken three orphan children, the oldest six years old, to look after, in addition to her own four, her mother, and her mother-in-law. There are no men left to do the work on the farm and poor Baquet did not know how they could get along. I gave him one hundred francs and told him it was from my friends in Canada. He did not want to take it at first, saying it was sent for the wounded, but I explained to him that it was sent to me to help the soldiers and the soldiers' families. He said it would mean so much to his wife, she works from four in the morning till dark. They are the sort of people who deserve help and it is such a joy to be able to lighten their burdens a little.

We have only about eighty patients at present, but they keep us busy. The two men who came in last have been so terribly wounded. We have had a number of cases of gas gangrene. They are trying to cure them with a new sort of serum. Two of the men really seem to be getting better. Four cases were brought in yesterday. One poor man died at noon and I was glad he did not live any longer; another they had to operate on in the afternoon and take his leg off. He was in very bad shape last night but this morning he surprised every one by asking for pen and paper to write to his mother, and says he feels fine.

Our wounded general left today. He could not say enough nice things about the hospital. He said he was so glad he had been brought here, not only on his own account, but he was so glad to see how wonderfully his men were taken care of.

The guns have been going incessantly for the past two days and we hear that the English have taken four trenches. I have also heard that some Canadians have come over lately and our Bayard may be only four or five miles from me. I asked the general if it would be possible for me to find out; he said he would inquire and if Bayard is anywhere in reach he would get me a pass to go and see him. I feel as if I would start out and walk to try and find him; but alas! one cannot get by the sentries without proper papers.

I hope my fur lined cape has not gone to the bottom. I think I shall still need it in June, for after two wonderful sunshiny days we are again freezing. Sunday and Monday were like days in June and we moved the beds of the patients out in the grass and others were on stretchers. We had the phonograph going, served lemonade, biscuits, sweets, and cigarettes. They had a wonderful time and all slept like tops the next night.

I think I shall have to find a new job when the war is over, for I don't think I shall ever do any more nursing.

I am trying to find a lot of straw hats like "cows' breakfasts" and cheap parasols to protect their heads when they are taking sun baths.

The dressings are taken down and one thickness of gauze only left over the wound, and they are left in the sun from twenty minutes to two hours according to what they can stand.

April 11, 1916

Yesterday we had quite an interesting time with aircraft. The machine came down so close, that we could see the pilot and his assistant who waved to us that they were going to throw something to us. A package landed, almost in the pond. It turned out to be a letter tied up in a handkerchief with some shot as weight. It was from the English boys who were patients here for a while; they told us they would pay us a visit some day. We could see the machine gun in front of the aeroplane quite distinctly. In the afternoon there was another excitement — a German machine chased by several French. It looked from below as if they had got him, but they all disappeared in the clouds and we did not know the result of the fight.

At nine o'clock there was a terrific explosion as if a bomb had dropped just outside the gate. We all rushed out and could hear the aeroplane distinctly, but could not see it; no damage was done near us. We have just heard that the bomb landed just outside the village doing no damage.

Thanks for the toilet articles, they are a wise selection. What we before considered necessities we now know are luxuries.

We have just got off a motor full of convalescents going home on permission. I hope they will get a month, some of them have been in the trenches twenty months.

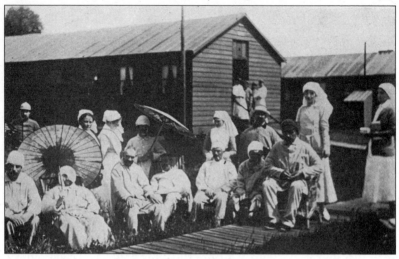

Showing linen caps and Chinese umbrellas. Purchased for patients
from contributions. *My Beloved Poilus*

May 3, 1916

I got a lot of linen hats and Chinese umbrellas to keep the sun off the
patients when they are out of doors.

The two Canadian nurses are a joy to work with, for they have had
splendid training and are the kind that will go till they drop. We have a
wounded German prisoner who was brought in three days ago. The poor
boy had to lose his right arm and was at first terrified of every one. He
expected to be ill-treated, but now that he sees he gets the same treatment
as all the other patients he is happy and contented and very glad to be with
us. I thought if I ever saw a German in these regions I would be capable
of killing him myself, but one cannot remember their nationality when
they are wounded and suffering.

I am sending you a photo of the Queen of the Belgians, who visited
us and was very nice; she spoke so highly of the Canadians and of the
splendid work they had done.

May 24, 1916
Paris

I left Dunkirk Thursday morning in time to escape the bombs, and stopped off at Étaples to look up some of our friends at the Canadian hospital. Dr. MacLaren had left for London but I saw Mary Domville and Dr. Margaret Parks.

Étaples is a real city of hospitals now. I saw the St. John Ambulance and the Canadian unit; they are both most interesting, so well organized.

Captain T____ took me to the station in a motor, for which I was glad, as it is two miles, and the walk over in the sun was as much as I wanted. Arrived at Paris at five the next morning rather weary, had a hot bath, the first in a real tub for eight months, and when I went to bed that night I slept for nearly twenty-four hours.

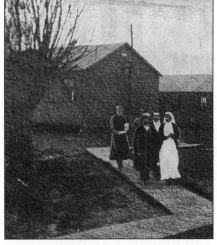

May 30, 1916
Divonne-les-Bains

I did not go to the Grand Hotel for reasons of economy. This is a clean little place and I am quite comfortable but I miss the bathroom and the balcony.

The Queen of the Belgians leaving the ambulance. *My Beloved Poilus*

There are no patients at the ambulance here for the moment. All the fighting is in the north and at Verdun. Poor Verdun — it is terrible there, one hundred days and still no let up — I think there will be no men left in France before long and then the English will have to take their turn. When will it all end? Divonne is as beautiful as ever, and so quiet and peaceful one would not realize that there was a war if it were not for the fathers and sons who will never come back, and the women who are struggling to make both ends meet. I have had news of several of my old patients who were here. Daillet, who was paralyzed, is at Vichy and can walk two miles with crutches, two others have been killed and many of the others back in the trenches. I have not been able to sleep, it is so quiet.

June 20, 1916
Mobile No. 1, France

Today I went over to Poperinghe to look up Margaret Hare. She is in charge of the Canadian clearing hospital and is doing a wonderful work. They have been getting all the wounded from this last fight — receive one day, evacuate the next, and the third day clean up and get ready again. It is wonderfully organized; the trains come right up to the hospital and there is a nurse for each car, so the patients are well looked after. Margaret has been mentioned in despatches, I believe. I am so glad, for she certainly deserves it.

June 25, 1916

I went over for Margaret Hare in the motor. She went with me to the cemetery near the hospital and I put some roses on the grave of one of our Saint John boys. I wish his mother could see how well cared for it is. Margaret came back to tea with us.

Today I have been specializing a man who has developed tetanus. I would almost wish that he would die, for he has no hands, and has a great hole in his chest and back, but strange to say he wants to live, is so patient and so full of courage. When I have cases like this one I am always so grateful to the people who have helped me in my work. If they could see the comforts that can be given by a bottle of cologne or a dozen oranges they would be rewarded.

Our medicine chef was a prisoner in Germany for eleven months. The things that he tells us makes one's blood boil. One cannot imagine human beings as brutal as the Germans are. When they came into the town where he had his hospital, they shot all the wounded that were left and eight of his orderlies who stayed with him. He expected to be shot also, but they needed his services so took him prisoner.

July 16, 1916

Another rainy day and as cold as the dickens, but we are glad to get through the summer without extreme heat or a pest of flies.

My tetanus case is really getting better.

Last week I went to a concert given at R___ for the soldiers who are resting. It was one of the nicest I have ever been at. I did not want to go, for I don't feel like any kind of gaiety, but Mrs. Turner insisted. There were only three ladies present, the rest of the *salle* was filled with soldiers just from the trenches. The concert was held in a stable.

Some English and Canadian officers, who are on construction work near here, have been coming to see us. One is Major H___, who was on the Courtenay Bay work at Saint John.

July 29, 1916

We are nearly eaten up with the mosquitoes so I have been to Dunkirk to get some mosquito netting.

Mrs. Turner gave a grand concert to the men on the anniversary of the opening of this hospital. Denries, from the *Opéra Comique* in Paris, and Madame Croiza, from the opera in Paris, sang. The Prince of Teck was here and in my ward, he was so nice to the patients. We had French, English, and Belgian generals, colonels, and officers of various kinds.

July 31, 1916
No. 3 Canadian Casualty Station

I got twenty-four hours permission and came out here to spend the night with Nursing Sister Margaret Hare, hoping to get some news of Bayard. I have found out where he is and that he has been on rest and went back to the trenches today. They are usually on duty eight days and off eight, so Margaret is going to send him word when he next comes off to come here and I will come over and meet him. I do hope we will be able to make [a] connection. It is so hard to be so near and yet not be able to see him. If he is wounded he will have to pass through No. 10 Clearing Station, which is right next to this. I have left my name and address at the office, so if he should be brought in they will telephone me and I can get over to him in half an hour. The patients here are so well taken care of. They have had a light day. I helped a little in the dressing room this morning, saw some of the men who had come in last night, saw three operations. There is a very clever English surgeon here and several McGill men. It is a scorching hot day.

My tetanus patient is quite cured, is beginning to walk about.

August 14, 1916
Mobile No. 1

We have had a strenuous and exciting week. It began with a visit from the King of the Belgians, who came to decorate three of my men who had fought in the trenches with conspicuous bravery. He visited all the wards and talked with the soldiers. Like all the royalty I have met so far, he is extraordinarily simple — wore no decorations or distinguishing marks of any kind. We were all presented to him in turn and shook hands with him.

The next day we got twenty gas cases and several badly wounded men — one Canadian from Ontario and two English boys, one was a policeman in London. I asked the Ontario man how he happened to get to our ambulance, he said, "he'd be blessed if he knew," he was working on the lines which run right up to the trenches when the warning for gas was given. He started to put on his helmet and the next thing he knew he was in a Red Cross ambulance on the way to the hospital. He is getting on splendidly but we lost four of the gas cases. It is the worst thing I have seen yet, much worse than the wounded, and the nursing is awfully hard, for they cannot be left a moment until they are out of danger.

August 28, 1916

I have met our boy Bayard at his rest camp not very far from here. It was a joy to find him looking so well, and big and brown.

September 9, 1916

Rain, continuous rain. The guns have been roaring without any let up for three days and nights, and our little barracks are nearly shaken to pieces. We have had several warnings of gas attacks, but fortunately nothing has happened. One of the orderlies kept his mask on all night and everyone was surprised that he was alive next morning, they are the most awful smelling things you can imagine.

We have never seen so many aeroplanes as during this past week. This morning we counted eighteen in a row.

Mrs. Turner is going to organize another hospital on the Somme and is going to keep this one as well. She certainly has done a splendid work. We are all hoping that the fighting will be over before Christmas.

October 1, 1916

The rain has begun, so I suppose we may expect to be under water for the rest of the winter, but things are going well for us, so we must hope on; but Oh! how dreadful it all is.

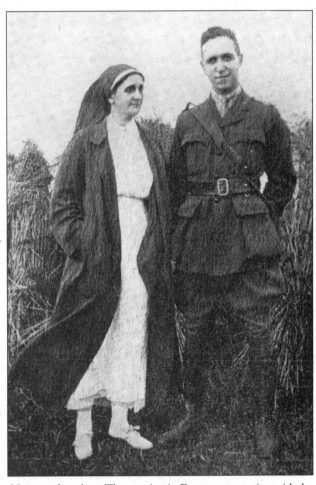

Nurse and nephew. The meeting in France, one serving with the
French, the other with the Canadian Expeditionary Force.

My Beloved Poilus

A stationary balloon that is not far from here, used as a Belgian observation post, was struck by a bomb from an aeroplane and we saw it fall in flames. The men who were in it jumped out with parachutes and both escaped without injury.

Broterl, the famous French sniper and poet, came the other day to sing for the soldiers. He is wonderful, and sang all sorts of songs that he had composed in the trenches. The men were enchanted, it does such a lot of good, for it makes them forget for a time.

One of our orderlies has just got word that one of his brothers has been killed at the Somme, another is dangerously wounded in the head, and a third has lost his leg — he has six brothers, all at the front.

One of the men in my ward got word of the death of his brother also. He was a stretcher bearer and was helping a German officer who was wounded. As soon as the German got to a place of safety he shot the poor man who had been helping him.

I am nearly frozen tonight and will have to go to bed.

October 9, 1916

Our Bayard has come through the Courcelette fight safely, where the New Brunswickers did such wonders; but Oh! at such a terrible cost.[7]

It has been very cold and rainy here. I am afraid the bad weather has set in.

Wish you would send me an aluminum hot water bottle for Christmas, another pair of Indian moccasins, and fill up the corners of the box with malted milk and maple sugar.

I shall never forget the poor little Breton who said when he saw me — as he roused a little when we were taking him from the ambulance — *maintenant je suis sauvé* (now I am saved).

I have just received a cheque from the Rothesay Red Cross. Since I

---

[7]   The 26th Battalion helped to capture the village of Courcelette, on the Somme, on September 15, 1916. During the attack it lost about 325 men.

began, my fund has never entirely given out, and I have been able to give such a lot of pleasure and comfort to the men.

If any one wants to know what to send me you might suggest Washington coffee like Lady T____ [Tilley?] sent. It was a great success.

I am too cold to write any more, so good-night.

I wish I had some of Maggie's crullers and squash pie, but the French don't know anything about squash pies.

Our poor man with a broken back has been moved to a hospital near his home so his family can see him. We sent him on a mattress, fixed up with pillows and cushions so that he did not suffer at all on the journey.

When I have anyone who is so ill as he was I bless the good people at home who have made it possible for me to give them what they need.

The guns are busy tonight, so I suppose we will be tomorrow.

November 12, 1916

I have not had any home letters for three weeks.

The 26th have a great reputation here and Saint John can be proud of them.

November 19, 1916

We have been shaken almost to pieces with vibrations from the guns these last three days. What must it be close at hand? On Wednesday we had a visit from the Taubes again. I could not sleep for the noise of the machines, so I went out to see what was happening. We could see the bombs dropping all around us, but fortunately none came very near.

November 26, 1916

How we laughed over your stories. Send us some more when you have them, anything to make us laugh. It is strange how one can laugh in spite of everything. I don't think we could live through it if it were not for the funny and foolish things that happen.

I got a letter from our boy today. It is such a relief to see the dirty little envelopes with the address in pencil. There is never much news, but just to know that he is alive is enough.

December 9, 1916

We have all been a little worried about Christmas this year, fearing that we should not be able to give the men a really good dinner. We have all been getting contributions and are turning them into the general fund, and now comes this fat cheque from the Canadian Red Cross at Saint John for my beloved *poilus*. How can I ever thank them enough for their generous gift! All anxiety on the dinner score is now removed. We have about two hundred and fifty, counting *infirmiers* and men that work about the hospital — they are soldiers who have been in the trenches for nearly two years, or been disabled through wounds or sickness, or exchanged prisoners from Germany unfit for military service. They call the hospital *le petit Paradis des blessés* and are so glad to be sent here. A man was brought in here the other day who was wounded for the second time, but he did not mind in the least about his wounds, he was so glad to get back. He is delighted because he will not be well enough to leave before Christmas.

We sent to England for some pop-corn, and today the men have been like a lot of happy children stringing the corn for the tree. They had never seen it before and were much interested. We made quite a successful popper out of a fly screen and a piece of wire netting.

The other night we were talking over the various experiences we have had since the beginning of the war — the terrible things we have seen — the sad stories we have heard, and the strange but very true friendships

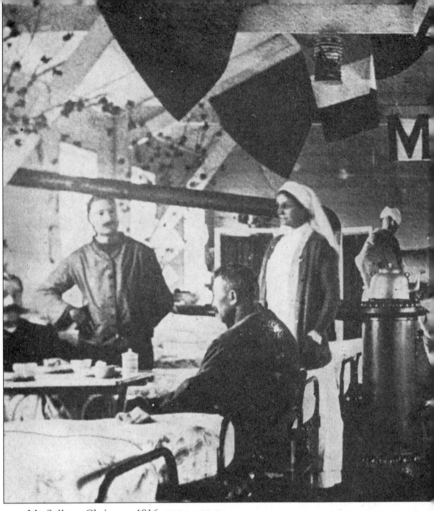

My *Salle* — Christmas 1916. *My Beloved Poilus*

we have formed — and we all agree that we could never have carried on our work in such a satisfactory way if it had not been for the gifts which have come from time to time from our home friends. The extra food that we have been able to give to the very sick men has made all the difference in the world to their recovery, and then the warm clothing when they go out, and the bit of money to help them over the hard place. You cannot imagine how much it means to them.

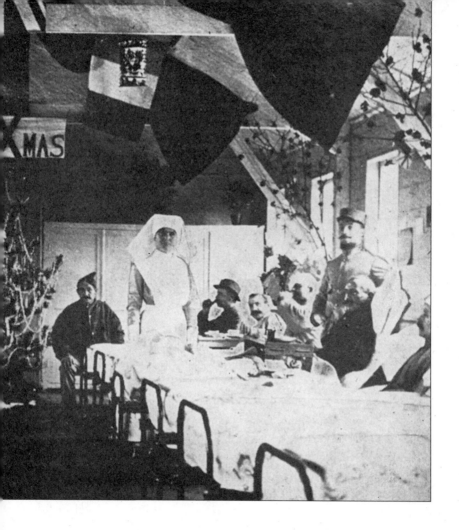

I remember so well one poor little man who had reached the limit of endurance, and when I found the sleepless nights were due to worry and not to pain, the whole pitiful little story came out. His wife was ill, his sister-in-law dead, and there were six children to be looked after — the eldest a boy of eleven — and no money. As long as his wife had been able to run the farm they had been able to get along, but she had given out. The French soldier only gets five cents a day, so he had nothing to send them. He cried like a baby when I told him I could help him. We sent off a money order for one hundred francs the next day, and I wish you could have seen the change in that man. That little sum of money put things straight six months ago and now everything is going well. But he will never forget, and both he and his wife have a very warm feeling in their hearts for the good people across the sea who came to their rescue in a time of need. When I begin to talk of my beloved French it is hard to stop.

January 1, 1917

The men had a wonderful Christmas day. They were like a happy lot of children. We decorated the wards with flags, holly, mistletoe, and paper flowers that the men made, and a tree in each ward. You cannot imagine how pretty they were. Each patient began the day with a sock that was hung to the foot of their bed by the night nurses. In each was an orange, a small bag of sweets, nuts, and raisins, a handkerchief, pencil, tooth brush, pocket comb and a small toy that pleased them almost more than anything else, and which they at once passed on to their children. They had a fine dinner — jam, stewed rabbit, peas, plum pudding, fruit, nuts, raisins, and sweets. The plum puddings were sent by the sister of one of the nurses.

In the afternoon the trees were lighted and we had the official visit of the medicine chef and all the staff. After the festivities were over we began preparing for the tree for the refugee children. We had thought that we would have enough left over to manage for fifty children, but the list grew to one hundred and twenty-five. The mayor of the village let us have a large room in his house, as the first place we had chosen was too small. We had the tree on Sunday afternoon and three hundred and thirty-one children arrived. Fortunately we had some extra things so there was enough of something to go around. They had a lovely time, each one got a small toy, a biscuit, and most of them a small bag of sweets and an orange. The oranges and sweets gave out, but there were enough biscuits and toys, but there was nothing left.

We are all dead tired, for we worked like nailers for the past two weeks; but it was worthwhile, for we were able to make a great many people happy, and now we are sending off packages to the trenches — things that came too late for Christmas.

We expect to move this month. It will be an awful business breaking up here, for all the barracks have to be taken to pieces and moved with us. We have begun to take an inventory and to pack up, but I do not know just where we will move to, the papers are not in order yet. It is hard to believe that another year of war has begun.

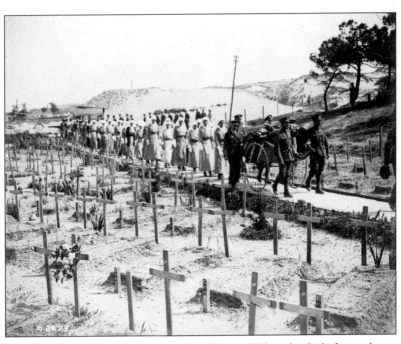

Funeral of Nursing Sister Gladys Maude Mary Wake, who died of wounds
received during a German air raid on Étaples, France, May 1918.

LAC-PA-002562

Chapter Five

After *My Beloved Poilus*

Nineteen seventeen picked up intensity where 1916 ended, bringing more responsibility for Warner, more critical cases, more patients, more danger. As the demands on her grew, it seemed impossible to get away, not even to be with her mother and siblings in Saint John when the sad news came that General D.B. Warner had passed away at the age of eighty-five. His obituary noted that his daughter Agnes was "nurse in charge of one of the important hospitals of the French Government on the Belgian Front."

That was February, and Warner was in the process of packing up and relocating Ambulance Mobile No. 1 to another part of Belgium. The ambulance would move several times again, always following the 36th Corps of the French army. Now expanded to hold more beds and handle more serious wounds closer to the front, the ambulance kept seventeen nurses on full-time duty. Warner took charge of this crew as the hospital's matron sometime before May 1917, just as the hazards of its work were multiplying. The *British Journal of Nursing* would caution in its May 26 issue that "The work at this hospital greatly appeals to the nurses, although the Matron, Miss Warner, carefully warns Sisters who wish to join the staff that they must be ready to put up with any difficulties."

"Difficulties" included working in noxious masks when mustard gas seeped into the hospital from the German lines and holding one's nerve through pounding air raids. Sometime in May or June, that nerve was severely tested when a German bomb fell directly on the hospital, injuring

Sister Jaffery's foot and producing fumes that rendered Sister Coppin unconscious when she rushed to save Jaffery. Matron Warner commended her staff for their "magnificent work under very dangerous conditions," like this bombing, which she always maintained was a deliberate attack on a clearly marked hospital. Indeed, in 1917 and 1918, reports of hospital bombings increased alongside bitter denouncements of German barbarism. Of the Canadian Army (C.A.M.C.) nurses alone, over forty-six lost their lives in bombings of Canadian hospitals and hospital ships, and posters vowing revenge further galvanized public resolve, most famously after the drowning death of fourteen nurses aboard the *Llandovery Castle*, including Anna Irene Stamers of Saint John, and the execution of British nurse Edith Cavell for helping Allied P.O.W.s escape from occupied Belgium. Nurses were largely beyond reproach in public opinion, and aggression against them provided the Allies with some of its most potent propaganda opportunities.

By mid-1917, *My Beloved Poilus* had been in press for several months and proceeds were reaching a grateful Warner. In May and June, *The Saint John Globe* published two responses to the book by Warner, the first written to an individual and the second meant for a wider group:

> The copy of *My Beloved Poilus* did not reach me until some time after I arrived here [at Ambulance Mobile No. 1]....I got the notification about the money from Messrs. Morgan, Harjes & Co. and they said the book which had been forwarded would explain it. I thought it was a book written by one of my friends, so I was quite unprepared for what came. I am very pleased that the book has sold, and am so glad to get the money for my men. We need more than ever here and I cannot expect people to keep on giving, when there are so many demands on every side. They have all been so good and generous to my *Poilus*. I shall write more fully about it very soon, but have not had a minute, there has been such a rush ever since we came....One poor man who has been awfully ill...says this is the first home he has

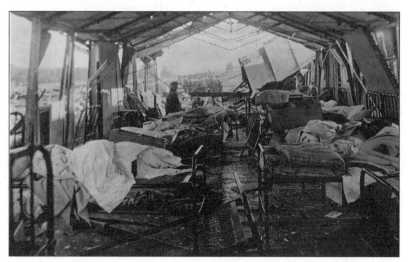

Bomb damage at a hospital. Queens University Archives

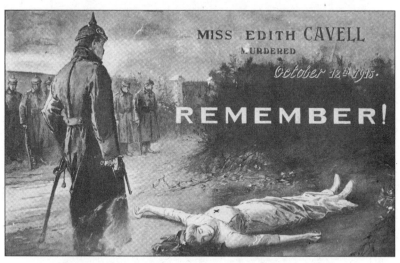

MISS EDITH CAVELL
MURDERED
October 12th 1915.

REMEMBER!

Propaganda poster of the execution of Nurse Edith Cavell.
CWM 19960034-008

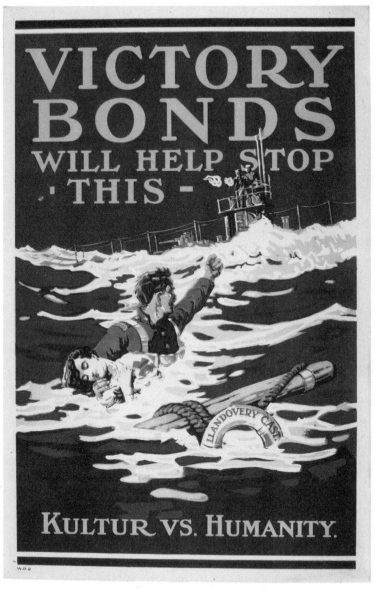

Propaganda poster depicting the German U-boat attack
on the Llandovery Castle. CWM 19850475-034

had since the war began. Just think of how he must have suffered to feel like that! His little girl is nearly three years old and he has never seen her — she was born after the war began. He adores Miss ___ — one of the Australian nurses who has been taking care of him. Fortunately, each one thinks his nurse is the best of the lot.

It is just as well you did not ask my consent before publishing the letters in *My Beloved Poilus*, for I never would have given it; and just think what a loss it would have been to my men!

How can I thank the friends and readers of "My Beloved Poilus" enough for all that they have done for me and my soldiers, and Mr. Cody for the very nice preface. Never in my wildest dreams would I have imagined that any one outside of the family would have been interested in my letters, and I can scarcely believe it is true that they have been the means of bringing in so much money. You have all been so good and kind about them and they have helped my *Poilus* so much. The state of one's mind and nerve at the end of a hard day is not conductive [*sic*] to good letter writing.

I am sending you the model of a Taube, the German aeroplane that has done so much bombarding. They are small and very swift and carry four, six or eight bombs. We see them very often, and the bombs drop too close to be pleasant sometimes. Yesterday a piece of shell went through the roof of one of our barracks, but fortunately no body was hurt....

[E]verything is going so well that we hope the war will be over before the end of the year. I do not see how it can last much longer.

The larrigans...arrived in time for Christmas and for

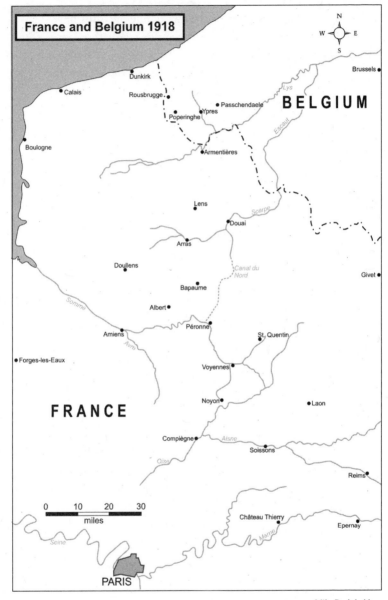

France and Belgium 1918

Brussels

Dunkirk
Rousbrugge
Passchendaele
BELGIUM
Calais
Poperinghe Ypres
Lys
Escaut
Boulogne
Armentières

Lens
Douai
Scarpe
Arras
Doullens
Givet
Canal du
Nord
Bapaume
Somme
Albert
Péronne
St. Quentin
Amiens
Avre
Forges-les-Eaux
Voyennes

FRANCE
Noyon
Laon

Compiègne
Aisne
Soissons
Oise

Reims

0 10 20 30
miles
Seine
Château Thierry
Marne
Epernay

PARIS

Mike Bechthold

the first time my feet were warm and dry in the terribly cold, wet, muddy weather we were having. Please thank many times all who were interested in sending me such a lovely present and one that would contribute so much to my comfort....

Over one thousand cases passed through this ambulance the first month we were here and before we were fully organized. Some stayed only twenty-four hours, but the badly wounded and the worst gas cases were kept. It was a great joy to have so many of them recover — when they first came in there did not seem to be much hope for them. We have sixteen nurses now, all well trained and such splendid women, it is a pleasure to work with them.

With heartfelt thanks to all,

THE WRITER OF THE POILUS LETTERS

❖

Warner had grown accustomed to packing the ambulance and moving it forward, but when the Germans launched a massive offensive in March 1918, Mobile No. 1 was evacuated and its staff sent to the interior. Facing a rapidly moving front line, authorities decided to position the hospital at a safe distance from the front, at Forges-les-Eaux, where it would function as a base hospital rather than an advanced ambulance. But within a couple months, Warner received this desperate letter from a doctor she had worked with for three years in Belgium. He was now serving at front-line ambulances associated with the 36th Corps and his plea was not subtle:

The wounded began to come at 23 o'clock, there were 600 in the yard, the rooms and the hall of our establishment. We worked all night hoping [for] some rest for the day after, but the arrivage was about 2,000 and every day like that during ten days. For five days Messr. R. (chief surgeon) and I were alone. We asked for you the first day. No compresses, no towels for the operations, amputations or debridgements. Extractions of projectiles were made on the *brancards* (stretchers) often without an anaesthetic. How many poor chaps died without care! How many would not be dead if you had been here! The evacuation was impossible. No trains, no motor cars. Oh, what an infinite suffering! Messr. R. is very very sorry, like me, to be deprived of your precious help.

The doctor's letter moved Warner and five other nurses immediately to request release from their current post so they could offer their services at the front. Authorization took three weeks. While they waited, she and Helen McMurrich worked in an overcrowded Paris hospital where for the first time Warner had the opportunity to care for American patients. She would later impress upon a Saint John audience the strength of the Americans' courage, their burning hatred for the enemy, and their bitter resentment at having shown up too "late" to the fight. For some of her listeners, this may well have been a new interpretation of the American position.

Not long after, Warner would be enthusiastically welcomed back among her old military and medical friends at an F.F.N.C. mobile hospital, Ambulance 16/21. Somehow, they found the wherewithal to celebrate·the reunion. Warner threw a Fourth of July party for the patients, with surprise bags for all, and the wards rang with shouts of "Vive l'Angleterre" and "Vive l'Amérique" as patients delivered a moving tribute to the nursing staff. (Warner, of course, was still identified as an American citizen, though primarily a resident of Canada.) Another summer night, convalescent patients and nurses took up the general's invitation to a theatrical performance, where Miss Warner took the seat of honour in the general's box and heard how badly she and the other sisters had been missed.

From that point on, the team of sisters learned to do even more, with even less. Nearly every three weeks they moved the ambulance from one pulverized part of France to another, looking for standing houses (three

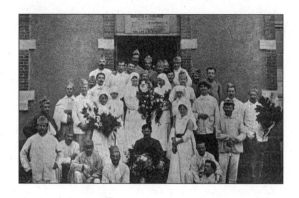

Nurses and staff of
Ambulance 16/21,
including Warner.
British Journal of Nursing

walls would do), factories, or chateaux that had survived the enemy's
scorched-earth practice and would be suitable for a temporary hospital, and
scavenging furnishings from empty houses. This time the nurses worked
closer to the front than ever. So many wounded men were lost in transit
over rough, muddy fields en route to the ambulance that at last it was
moved forward to a point just ten kilometres from the front line. Without
the necessary surgical supplies, "we could only save fifty per cent," Warner
would later tell a Saint John reporter, "but we did all we could, and the
men knew that and they were not left alone."

Just as the soldiers daily transcended their most basic fears in the face
of mortal danger, so the nurses of Ambulance 16/21 steeled their own
nerves. When the lights went out and the bombardments came, nurses
steadily made their rounds in the dark, heedless of their patients' pleas to
"Lie down on the ground, Sister, it's safer that way." One sister woke in the
night to the shock of a bomb's force blowing out one side of the house in
which she was sleeping, and "on being told it was only the other side of the
house and not the walls immediately above her, she went to sleep again."

The workload was crushing and hazardous, but with the Allies'
counterattack pushing the German line steadily back, Warner could finally
dare to predict the end of the conflict. Ten days before the Armistice she
wrote:

> The pressure of work has been terrific, but we are having a
> let up now, and the rest of our staff has joined us, so it will

not be so hard. We are not much to look at these days, but we can work. The washing is an awful problem....

[T]he rain has started in...but so far we have had enough fuel to keep the stoves going. The holes in our house have been patched up and the windows pasted over with paper where the glass is missing, so we feel that we are in luxury, being able to keep both dry and warm. We are in St. Quentin and living in the remains of a real house....

In each of our bedrooms we have small stoves that we found in the houses about here; whatever we needed in the way of furniture, we got from the ruined houses or from the streets or from the trenches nearby. Most of the things had to be mended, for what the Boches did not take away with them they destroyed. However, this place has escaped better than some of the others we have been in, for they did not have time to do their work as thoroughly as they usually do. Unfortunately the beautiful old church of the twelfth century is a mass of ruins. I think we are getting very near the end, and if peace is not signed before Christmas, at least the fighting will be over. Three of the Australian nurses are leaving Mobile No. 1 to return home. They were most anxious to join us, but feared the life would be too hard for Miss S___, who had about come to the end of her tether.

The hospital is in tents; we have three tents with twenty-four beds in each, so it keeps me going.

We were the first nursing unit to cross the Hindenburg line as far as I know, at least the first French one.

I have been on night duty for three weeks and have one more week to go.

I have had many interruptions while writing this letter, and now must put it away to begin my morning work, as it is 5 a.m.

We do not know how Warner and the others of Ambulance 16/21 observed the Armistice. If they were privy to the war news, they would have known by the beginning of November that the end was imminent, and any elation they might have felt about the formalities of November 11 must have been swallowed by immediate realities demanding the same full-on effort as they'd given the day before, and the days before that. For Warner, the Armistice ushered in "perhaps the saddest sights of the whole war": civilian prisoners formerly kept in concentrated labour camps, now released in shocking condition, vermin-infested, exhausted, emaciated, "stagger[ing] to the thresholds of their own homes." As far west as Givet, Warner's unit cared for these former prisoners as their final act of mercy in a four-and-a-half-year mission. Then the cosmopolitan little group disbanded and each prepared to go home.

They returned exhausted but triumphant. They also returned decorated. Warner herself had been twice mentioned in despatches and wore three important French military awards, including the *Médaille d'Honneur* in Bronze, awarded March 29, 1917, by the French minister of war to the *Infirmière Major* of Mobile No. 1 "for her zeal and devotion. In order to perpetuate in her family, and in the midst of her fellow citizens the memory of her honourable conduct." On December 1, 1917, Warner was given the special honour reserved for courageous life-saving actions: the *Médaille des Épidémies — L'Insigne Spécial en Or*, for the assiduous care and devotion she lavished on sick and wounded soldiers throughout the war.

On December 1, 1918, the entire unit of Ambulance 16/21 received a special letter of commendation and praise from General Nollet, commander of the 36th Corps, for its superb efficiency and effort in providing military and civilian care at Givet during the final weeks of the war. Another prestigious honour came just prior to Warner's fourth Christmas on the continent. The *British Journal of Nursing* presented a full account of the event in its January 4, 1919, issue:

> On December 20st, the General of the 36ème Corps d'Armée sent an order to say that he wished to come and decorate the Sisters of the Ambulance 16/21.

On December 21st, the Inspector of the *Service de Santé* of the 36ème Corps sent an order to have all the orderlies and stretcher-bearers lined up for inspection, previous to the decoration of the *Infirmières Anglaises*, and that all was to be in readiness by 2 p.m. that day.

It was not easy to find a suitable spot, as the ambulance is "en repos" in a remote little straggling village; but finally it was decided to fix on a field opposite the Sisters' "messroom," and there the men were lined up. At 2 p.m. the Inspector arrived and reviewed the men, and at 2:30 the General arrived. The Sisters had been told where to stand. After the review of the men they were called up to stand facing the General, and with them was one of the Aumoniers of the corps. The General read out the citations and pinned on the *Croix de Guerre*, after each citation he told each Sister what pleasure he had in presenting her with the decoration which she had so well-earned.

Before he pinned the medal to Warner's uniform, the general read the following citation in French: "Miss Warner (Agnes Louise). Infirmière Major, Ambulance 16/21, has been in the 'formations sanitaires' of the French Armies for four years, where she is well-known as a model of enduring energy, of disinterestedness and of devotion. Spent day and night attending to gassed and severely wounded cases, regardless of fatigue and bombardments. Has commanded the admiration of all."

Besides Agnes Warner, Sisters Annie Mildred Hanning, Helen McMurrich, and Mabel Constance Jones received the *Croix de Guerre* on this day for their acts of heroism and courage. It was a meaningful award for these sisters who had seen their adored *poilus* thus decorated on several occasions. Few women received this award in the First World War and even fewer foreign women, but several of those who did were F.F.N.C. nurses.

With Canadian Sister Helen McMurrich, Agnes Warner had worked, rested, and travelled since they first met in 1916, and now they shared the journey home together on the *Rochambeau* out of Le Havre. The liner docked in New York on February 28, 1919, and that week the Saint John papers heralded Warner's imminent return to the city. But she would not reappear in Saint John for fully a month. The reason, according to her closest friends, was that the physical demands of her final tour through the wasteland beyond the Hindenburg Line took more from an exhausted Warner than she could spare. Her strength gave way to an unspecified illness — perhaps something tenacious she had been exposed to in the sick wards of France. The setback compelled her to stay on Long Island with her former clients and steady supporters, the Eldridges, until "somewhat renewed" in health, and while there she probably sought treatment at the Presbyterian Hospital. Warner was not a young woman. She had joined the F.F.N.C. pushing the upper limit of its eligible age range and by the end of the war she was in her mid-forties.

Warner's stayover in New York gave the Saint John devotees time to prepare an ambitious welcome home. Her sisters and brother John, along with enthusiastic members of the I.O.D.E. (De Monts Chapter) met her at the train on March 29 and whisked her into a whirl of receptions, teas, and tributes at which she was not only the guest of honour but the keynote speaker as well.

First, the Royal Standard Chapter of the I.O.D.E. had its turn, presiding over a studio festooned with flags, bunting, and flower arrangements in red, white, and blue. One lady had the vision to place a flag of France "most artistically so that it seemed to mount guard over Miss Warner and to appreciate its privilege of caring for one who had done so much for La Belle France." It must have struck a grand emotion to hear the orchestra play *God Save the King*, *The Star Spangled Banner*, *Rule Britannia*, *O Canada*, and "with most impressive effect, the glorious music of the *Marseillaise*." Soloist Miss McKnight moved the audience with the touching First World War ode to nurses, "The Rose of No Man's Land," and other contemporary hymns to peace and victory. On account of her Belgian heritage, Mrs. D. Mullin was selected to present the address:

After four years of heroic self sacrifice, untold hardships and unswerving devotion to the noble cause of humanity, you the daughter of that distinguished general...have returned to the land of your childhood — this Canada of ours — to enjoy a well merited rest from your arduous labors. Yes, after four years of patient, gratuitous toil among your beloved poilus, to whom you were as a ministering angel alleviating the sufferings of their sick and wounded, regardless of the attendant discomforts ever surrounding you, you have come back to us decorated with every distinction that France could bestow. Yet were the Recording Angel to ask concerning your works of mercy that which you desired he should set down in his "Book of Gold," notwithstanding the distinguished honors conferred upon you, we feel you would adapt the words of Abou Ben Adhem, who said: "Write me as one who loved his fellow men."

Not surprisingly, Warner's reply deftly shifted the accolades where she felt they were more appropriately due.

[She] thanked the chapter for the occasion and the gift saying that she had done no more than many other nurses and had felt it a great privilege to be able to do her part. She said that she had often heard that men cannot bear suffering as can women but she could never agree to this since she had seen her wounded Poilus suffer such unbelievable things with courage, fortitude, endurance and resignation in order that freedom and liberty might prevail.

How she must have struggled to describe these unknown soldiers with their unseen wounds to friends who could never fully visualize endless mud-caked, blistered, bleeding bodies. How her audience must have struggled to understand what it was like to internalize that dreadful responsibility for so many lives. But, by implicit contract, both parties expressed themselves in glorious superlatives rather than gritty realities, leaving most of the "unbelievable things" locked in the minds of Agnes and others like her who could never forget them.

When Warner did relate her experience, it was in rolling narrative, with the air of an adventure story. On April 7, she spoke to a group of one hundred and fifty members of the Women's Canadian Club gathered for another lavish reception in her honour. Several other Saint John nursing sisters were present (most of them C.A.M.C.), although club president Mrs. Kuhring regretted that it had not been possible to invite *all* of the area nursing sisters, only those who had received decorations. She stood to thank the nurses who had "given these examples of great womanhood and gone where others could not go to care for in the most minute way those precious bodies which meant so much to those at home." Then she introduced the guest of honour. In its report on the occasion, the Saint John *Standard* noted: "On rising to speak, Nursing Sister Warner, who was greeted with prolonged applause, said that she thanked all present for the honor but that she had only done what the other sisters did." Then Warner went on to give highlights of her movements through Divonne and later Belgium.

> At one hospital where Miss Warner was they took the
> badly wounded cases who could not go any farther, but
> who would have died without the care the nurses were
> able to give them. The speaker here paid a high tribute
> to the work of the French surgeons and French priests....
> They were at first inclined to be suspicious of the
> sisters, asking what these foreign women who were not
> "religious" were doing there, but a Franciscan monk who
> had been nine years in Montreal said, "Wait and see,"
> and soon they were the best of friends and worked
> together caring for the men.
>
> There was a Church of England clergyman, an
> ambulance driver, who sometimes could hold a service

but at other times the sisters went to the Roman Catholic services held in a little chapel made of wood just big enough for the priest, while the people remained in the road....

The winter of 1917 was the coldest one, and there was no fuel to be had, everybody was cold except the patients, and the sisters would often go out and gather up sticks. A Belgian sentry used to give them a few bags of coal and these were repaid by smokes and comforts. Near this place was a Canadian Engineers' camp, and Miss Warner told of Capt. Morrison's ruse to meet with the sisters and share their tea. Once while the sisters were having tea a general came to the hospital and asked for Mrs. Turner. Miss Warner talked with this visitor and he seemed so disappointed at not finding Mrs. Turner, and knowing there would be no tea nearer than Dunkirk she invited him to stay. Introducing the nurses, Miss Warner realized that she did not know the guest's name, but knew from his ribbons that his distinctions were many, and on inquiring he answered "Prince Alexander of Teck." Miss Warner said she got weak in the knees, but he was very nice and came to see them several times. He was the British representative in the Belgian Government.

The report in the *Standard* continued:

Speaking of the air raids of which many occurred Miss Warner said she did not hold with the theory that when hospitals were bombed it was accidental. The planes came near enough to see the black crosses on them so it was clear the Germans could see the red crosses on the hospitals. Once a nurse had half her foot taken off and several times patients were injured while in their beds. The raids were frightful.

Many and pathetic were the stories told of the men. One big Scotchman came in shell shocked and very violent. On being given a hot cup of Washington coffee, and spoken to in English he came to himself. "You are among friends and quite safe," Miss Warner told him, and asked what he wanted. "My mither," he said. "That was always the cry," Sister Warner went on to say, "English, French or Canadian, and it was our privilege to take the mother's place as far as we could." The Washington coffee made with a fire of solidified alcohol had saved many lives and the stream of it had never ceased.

At one hospital the Americans were met with and their general feeling seemed to be of resentment that they had not been allowed to come sooner. "We got here a bit late but we've got to do our damndest," one westerner said.

Supplying their hospital from the trenches abandoned by the Germans, a stove which they were just going to light was found to be full of hand grenades, and Miss Warner said it made her blind with rage to see the wanton destruction everywhere. The cruel treatment of the children in the conquered areas was another description which made her hearers feel the horrors of the Huns and the state of the prisoners who reached the French hospital was indescribably pathetic.

The report concluded:

Speaking of the soldiers, Miss Warner told of the care they took of the sisters who were all alone on the French front but went everywhere with perfect safety and without any fear. "Make all excuses for the men," she said. "We have seen them at their best, patient, uncomplaining, thinking only of others. No one, except those who were there can realize what the men did. They were wonderful. Don't spoil them, give them work but count nothing too much to do for them. Wash off the mud, and you'll find the pure gold. We sisters can never be grateful enough for being allowed to help."

Three days later, a "thronged house" of Saint John High School alumnae heard another account, reported in the *Daily Telegraph*:

Of the patients' field hospital to which she went after the first year of the war Miss Warner told many wonderful things... of the boy field telephonist who thought his oxygen treatment was more telephoning, and said as he died that God was at the other end of the line; and of the orderlies drawn from all ranks and classes, twenty-seven of them priests, and some more intellectual than practical, even to the extent of using cocoa instead of a cleanser to scrub a table.

Miss Warner described the King and Queen of Belgium as she had seen them when they visited this field hospital. The queen had inadvertently been shown Miss Warner's own room which as it was used as the storeroom for supplies from home was more useful than tidy and was known as "The High Class Bazaar." The king, she said, was keenly interested in flying and often flew over the hospital.

The gifts sent from St. John had been of untold worth in emergencies especially, Miss Warner said, and the money from the book of her letters published by George Cushing had, she said, been put to such excellent use that she had almost forgiven him for publishing it. One of the pictures which she showed at the close of her address was of two patients wearing De Monts Chapter dressing gowns.... [S]he was able to assure the audience that all supplies they had sent would be put to good use as any

that remained are now being distributed to the refugees
and returned prisoners.

The report added:

Miss Warner had afterwards accompanied the ambulance
that followed the 36th regiment [sic] through the
devastated regions around St. Quentin. She told of the
hurried marches through the dreary land where sign posts
said of a heap of ruins that before the war this was such
and such a place. She described the venturesome journeys
for supplies returning by darkness through a wilderness
of mud and shell holes; and told also of the joys in
one French village retaken after four years of German
suppression where French flags had been unearthed from
their burying places and the people welcomed their own
grey clad soldiers for the first time, never having seen the
French uniform.

Of the scarcity of all materials and how the inhabitants
contrived to do without she told many strange tales. A
spool of thread was valued at $4 in one village and the
children saw cows for the first time after the Germans
were driven from the town. The devilish cruelty of the
Germans was illustrated by Miss Warner in several
forcefully told stories.

She appealed to her hearers in conclusion not to
think that now the war was over France needed no more
help. Her soldiers were not being welcomed as ours are.
They were returning to desolate homes. Thousands of
her villages were more desolate than Halifax after the
explosion and many men knew not whether their families
were alive or dead. For our own returning men she asked
that they be dealt with patiently for they had endured
almost the impossible. While at the front there was

nothing that was not noble; in the idleness of inaction at the rear there must be discontent and trouble. There were two forms of vision, she said. [Of] two men looking from the same window one would see mud and the other stars. The stars were there if they were only looked at and even in the mud of Flanders the nurses had seen them reflected brightly.

Warner's defence of soldiers' conduct holds an interesting hint that her audience had been exposed to media reports over the course of the war tarnishing popular images of military chivalry. This appeal for leniency coming from the irreproachable figure of a nurse was a powerful endorsement, and she seized this public opportunity to offer it as well as to reassert the "devilish cruelty" of the enemy. In her lectures, she made a point of contrasting very "feelingly" the essential nobility of one side with the demonstrated depravity of the other. Did this conviction come from reflecting on the debased behaviour that she witnessed, including even her own patients' enthusiasm for violence? As she bent over dressings and listened to her *poilus* boast about how they had routed the enemy, did a peaceable nurse from Saint John require a comparative morality to come to terms with the ugly actions of both sides without sliding into a paralyzing relativism? She was now reassuring others as she had herself: that the enemy perpetrated the greater inhumanity — and more gratuitously.

❖

As a lifetime achievement, nursing in the War to End All Wars was a tough act to follow. The day-to-day intensity and personal growth could not be matched by anything in the nurses' experience before or after. Gripped by the awful thought that the rest of her life would be nothing more than a denouement, an F.F.N.C. colleague of Agnes Warner's lamented: "Alas! I have said farewell to the most interesting period of my life. Never before have I, a plain and poor person, been able to realize myself. . . . I do hope I don't shrivel up again when they no longer need me." Another affirmed: "This great responsibility, and closeness with tragedy, seem to have started one off growing again....I really am a bigger person, humanly speaking." Alert, independent, and confident from their time at the front, these women were reluctant to trade the passion of emergency for the stifling confines of routine. They worried that they would soon tire of regular nursing.

Continuing as a military nurse was not an option, since army authorities reduced the C.A.M.C. to its pre-war size, retaining just a handful of permanent nurses. But there were new opportunities to be seized in the nursing field. The influenza pandemic of 1918 required many health-care hands, and great numbers of returning veterans needed the professional service of nurses trained in physiotherapy to help them reintegrate into work and family life. New spaces for travelling public health nurses and mental health nurses reflected changing societal attitudes about public health education and mental illness, while positions in schools and health centres with the Red Cross and the maturing Victorian Order of Nurses

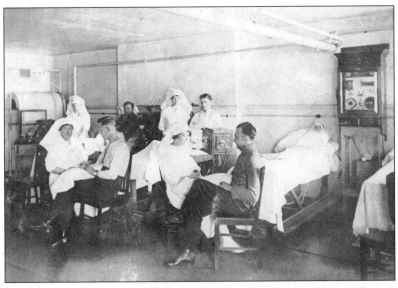

Nurses and patients at the Physiotherapy Department, New Brunswick Military Hospital, Fredericton. NBM1990.11.78

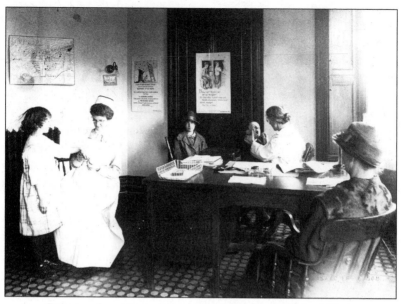

Doctor and nurse examining several children at the School Clinic
at the Saint John Health Centre. NBM NANB-SJHealthCentre-pg8

(V.O.N.) occupied a greater number of nurses than ever before. By 1921,
the number of nurses in Canada had more than tripled from a decade
before. Many of them were demobilized military nurses trying out a new
sub-vocation in one of these developing fields.

The extent to which the war was a catalyst for greater gender equality
even as it summoned a powerful impulse to reinstate "comfortable"
pre-war conditions, including traditional gender roles, is still a matter of
debate. True, many women had contributed to their nation's war effort
by filling factory and farm positions in the absence of men, proving they
could perform effectively in male-dominated roles. But now these same
women left their posts to returning veterans and many went back to their
firesides. In the relief and chaos that followed the Armistice, it became
clear that wartime changes would be considered a temporary aberration;
that women on the homefront had been encouraged to act in the place of
men only "for the duration." And women at the battlefront had not been

welcomed into male roles at all, but were restricted to non-combat roles as nurses, aides, and clerks. Ultimately, though women's wartime service and bravery may have helped to "earn" them the vote (in the rhetoric of the day), it did little to augment materially their social and political power or to weaken the polarity of separate spheres in the postwar decade.

For Warner, who returned from the war in questionable health, like so many of her beloved *poilus*, a full-time career in nursing was likely out of the question; so, now in her late forties, she entered semi-retirement. Thereafter, she kept busy with "missionary activity" (possibly volunteer work) with the Saint John Health Centre and cared for her aging mother in their South End home at 11 Pagan Place. She also corresponded faithfully with many of her former French patients and their families, sharing a unique bond with them that only battlefront initiates could truly fathom.

Sister Warner would live only seven more years. Her final trip to New York was to seek treatment at the Presbyterian Hospital for the most serious phase of the unnamed illness that still afflicted her. Sadly, there was little her *alma mater* could do to restore her, and she succumbed to the illness on April 23, 1926. Arrangements were made to carry her remains back to Saint John, and the following stormy Sunday a large congregation gathered for a heroine's funeral at Trinity Anglican Church and final farewells at Fernhill Cemetery.

❖❖

Aside from the brief, obligatory lecture circuit when she landed back in Saint John and the periodic wartime letters that kept family and friends apprised of her work, there was no evidence that Warner continued to process her wartime experiences with a view to publishing them. On the contrary, eulogizers praised her "modesty" in keeping silent about her overseas achievements, declaring that "at no time has she said a great deal of the life she endured." In reality, conditions in New Brunswick after the war probably did not invite a frank recollection of what happened or any attempt to grapple with its rawness. Acquaintances who had spent the war on Canadian soil may have been willing and eager confidantes, but they lacked the terrible literacy of front-line work that the nurses now carried. And others who themselves had returned from overseas carried their own unique experiences and processed each memory differently. In the postwar world, it is hardly surprising that so many nurses pulled a screen across their war work in order to get on with their interrupted lives and forge a "new normal." It is even less surprising that they kept silent about what they encountered near the front. Moreover, many nurses must have internalized the persistent ideal of selfless "modesty" that applauded a woman for claiming nothing particularly important about her own experience. Were it not for Agnes Warner's friends promoting the letters on her behalf, Saint John and the wider world might never have discovered a New Brunswick nurse's faithful service to countless families, nor had the opportunity to be humbled by the boundless compassion she showed her beloved *poilus*.

Acknowledgements

I first encountered Nurse Agnes Warner's remarkable story as part of a project initiated by Lianne McTavish, for which I was investigating the contributions of women to the New Brunswick Museum in the late nineteenth century. At that time, Dr. Stephen Clayden, Head of Botany and Mycology at the N.B.M. introduced me to Warner's exceptional collection of botanical specimens, pointed to her intriguing book of First World War letters, and generously shared what he had uncovered about Warner and her family. I am so grateful to him for that introduction to Miss Warner and for encouraging me to dig deeper into her life.

Thanks to Marc Milner for expanding the scope of the project and connecting me with the New Brunswick Military Heritage Project, thereby launching this glimpse into the great work of our province's nursing sisters. I am very grateful to Marc and to Brent Wilson for answering questions and facilitating the project through many phases. Special thanks to Brent, who patiently edited the manuscript, obtained the images, coordinated all input, and handled dozens of other tasks prior to publication. I'm grateful to Mike Bechthold for creating the maps that follow Nurse Warner's path through France and Belgium. Doug Knight and Susan Ross of the Canadian War Museum assisted in obtaining photos. And I owe many thanks to the staff at Goose Lane Editions for their editorial and design expertise.

For his impeccable judgment and serene endurance, I thank Greg Quinn, without whose advice and encouragement this project would have languished. And finally, I remember with appreciation every heartening word from family and friends who took an interest in this undertaking.

Selected Bibliography

Adami, J. George. *War Story of the Canadian Army Medical Corps.*
London: Colour Ltd., 1918. Available online at: http://digital.library.
upenn.edu/women/adami/camc/camc.html

Anonymous. *Mademoiselle Miss: Letters from a First World War Nurse at
an Army Hospital near the Marne.* Cornwall: Diggory Press, 2006.
Originally published 1916, Macmillan.

British Journal of Nursing, volumes 53-62 (1914-1919). Available online
at: http://rcnarchive.rcn.org.uk/ and http://www.archive.org/search.
php?query=british%20journal%20of%20nursing%20AND%20
collection%3Atoronto

Bruce, Constance. *Humour in Tragedy: Hospital Life behind 3 Fronts by a
Canadian Nursing Sister.* London: Skeffington, 1918.

The Canadian Nurse, volumes 10-11 (1914-1915). Available online at:
http://www.archive.org/search.php?query=the%20canadian%20
nurse Hallett, Christine E. "The Personal Writings of First World
War Nurses: A Study of the Interplay of Authorial Intention and
Scholarly Interpretation," *Nursing Inquiry* 14 (4, 2007): 320-329.

Higonnet, Margaret R., ed. *Nurses at the Front: Writing the Wounds of the
Great War.* Boston: Northeastern University Press, 2001. Includes
two primary texts: Ellen N. La Motte, *The Backwash of War* (New
York: G.P. Putnam's Sons, 1916); and Mary Borden, *The Forbidden
Zone* (New York: Doubleday, 1929, 1930).

Higonnet, Margaret Randolph, Jane Jenson, Sonya Michel, and
Margaret Collins Weitz, eds. *Behind the Lines: Gender and the Two
World Wars.* New Haven, CT and London: Yale University Press,
1987.

Macphail, Andrew. *Official History of the Canadian Forces in the Great War 1914-19: The Medical Services*. Ottawa: F.A. Acland, 1925. Available in print or online at: http://www.archive.org/details/medicalservices00macpuoft

Mann, Susan. *Margaret Macdonald: Imperial Daughter*. Montreal and Kingston, ON: McGill-Queen's University Press, 2005.

————, ed. *The War Diary of Clare Gass 1915-1918*. Montreal and Kingston, ON: McGill-Queen's University Press, 2000.

————. "Where Have All the Bluebirds Gone? On the Trails of Canada's Military Nurses, 1914-1918," *Atlantis* 26 (1, 2001): 35-43.

Morton, Desmond. *When Your Number's Up: The Canadian Soldier in the First World War*. Toronto: Random House, 1993.

Nicholson, G.W.L. *Canada's Nursing Sisters*. Toronto: Stevens, 1975.

Quiney, Linda. "Assistant Angels: Canadian Voluntary Aid Detachment Nurses in the Great War," *Canadian Bulletin of Medical History* 15 (1, 1998): 189-206.

Scott, Eric, ed. *Nobody Ever Wins a War: The World War I Diaries of Ella Mae Bongard, R. N.* Ottawa: Janeric Enterprises, 1998.

Smith, Angela K. *The Second Battlefield: Women, Modernism and the First World War*. Manchester, UK: Manchester University Press, 2000.

Stuart, Meryn. "War and Peace: Professional Identities and Nurses' Training, 1914-1930," in *Challenging Professions: Historical and Contemporary Perspectives on Women's Professional Work*, edited by Elizabeth Smyth, Sandra Acker, Paula Bourne, and Alison Prentice. Toronto: University of Toronto Press, 1999.

Veterans Affairs Canada. *Canada's Nursing Sisters*. Ottawa, 2005. Available online at: http://www.vac-acc.gc.ca/content/history/other/Nursing/nursingsister_eng.pdf

Warner, Agnes. *My Beloved Poilus*. Saint John, NB: Barnes & Co., 1917.

Wilson-Simmie, Katherine M. *Lights Out! A Canadian Nursing Sister's Tale*. Belleville, ON: Mika, 1981.

Web pages and Virtual Exhibitions:

Canadian War Museum. "Canada and the First World War." Available at: http://www.warmuseum.ca/cwm/exhibitions/guerre/home-e.aspx

Library and Archives Canada. "The Call to Duty: Canada's Nursing Sister." Available at: http://www.collectionscanada.gc.ca/nursing-sisters/index-e.html

New Brunswick Museum. *"Mark Our Place": World War I*. Virtual Exhibit. Available at: http://website.nbm-mnb.ca/MOP/english/ww1/index.asp

Veterans Affairs Canada. "Canada Remembers." Available at: http://www.vac-acc.gc.ca/remembers/

Photo Credits

The photos on the front cover (top) (LAC-PA-002562) and bottom (LAC-PA-006783), pages 9 (LAC-PA-5230), 25 (LAC 1970-163), and 128 (LAC-PA-002562) appear courtesy of Library and Archives Canada (LAC). The drawing on page 11 appeared in the book *Humour in Tragedy*. The photos on pages 14 (19920085-102), 20 (19920044-811), 22 (19590034-002), posters on pages 30 (19920143-009) and 39 (19900076-809), photos on pages 56 (19720102-061), 59 (19920085-529), the bottom photo on page 131 (19960034-008), and the photo on page 132 (19850475-034) and back cover (19700046-012 — illustration; and 19590034-002 — uniform) appear courtesy of the Canadian War Museum (CWM). The photo on pages 18 and 19 (V28 Mil-Hosp-10) appears courtesy of Queen's University Picture Collection. The posters on pages 21 (WP1.F12.F2) and 49 (WP1.B12. F2) appear courtesy of McGill University. The photos on pages 34 and 35 (1990.11.4), 36 (NANB-Military-7), 44 (VP-02816), 149 (1990.11.78), and 150 (NANB-SJHealthCentre-pg8) appear courtesy of the New Brunswick Museum (NBM). The photos on pages 40, 53, 69, 73, 75, 93, 95, 104, 108, 114, 115, 120, 124-125, and photo of Agnes Warner on back cover from *My Beloved Poilus*. The maps on pages 47, 52, and 134 appear courtesy of Mike Bechthold. The top photo on page 131 appears courtesy of the Queens University Archives. The photo on page 137 appears courtesy of the *British Journal of Nursing*. All illustrative material is reproduced by permission.

Index

The New Brunswick Military Heritage Project

The New Brunswick Military Heritage Project, a non-profit organization devoted to public awareness of the remarkable military heritage of the province, is an initiative of the Brigadier Milton F. Gregg, VC, Centre for the Study of War and Society of the University of New Brunswick. The organization consists of museum professionals, teachers, university professors, graduate students, active and retired members of the Canadian Forces, and other historians. We welcome public involvement. People who have ideas for books or information for our database can contact us through our website: www.unb.ca/nbmhp.

One of the main activities of the New Brunswick Military Heritage Project is the publication of the New Brunswick Military Heritage Series with Goose Lane Editions. This series of books is under the direction of Marc Milner, Director of the Gregg Centre, and J. Brent Wilson, Publications Director of the Gregg Centre at the University of New Brunswick. Publication of the series is supported by a grant from the Canadian War Museum.

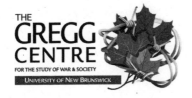

The New Brunswick Military Heritage Series

Volume 1

Saint John Fortifications, 1630-1956, Roger Sarty and Doug Knight

Volume 2

Hope Restored: The American Revolution and the Founding of New Brunswick, Robert L. Dallison

Volume 3

The Siege of Fort Beauséjour, 1755, Chris M. Hand

Volume 4

Riding into War: The Memoir of a Horse Transport Driver, 1916-1919, James Robert Johnston

Volume 5

The Road to Canada: The Grand Communications Route from Saint John to Quebec, W.E. (Gary) Campbell

Volume 6

Trimming Yankee Sails: Pirates and Privateers of New Brunswick, Faye Kert

Volume 7

War on the Home Front: The Farm Diaries of Daniel MacMillan, 1914-1927, ed. Bill Parenteau and Stephen Dutcher